The Curated Closet

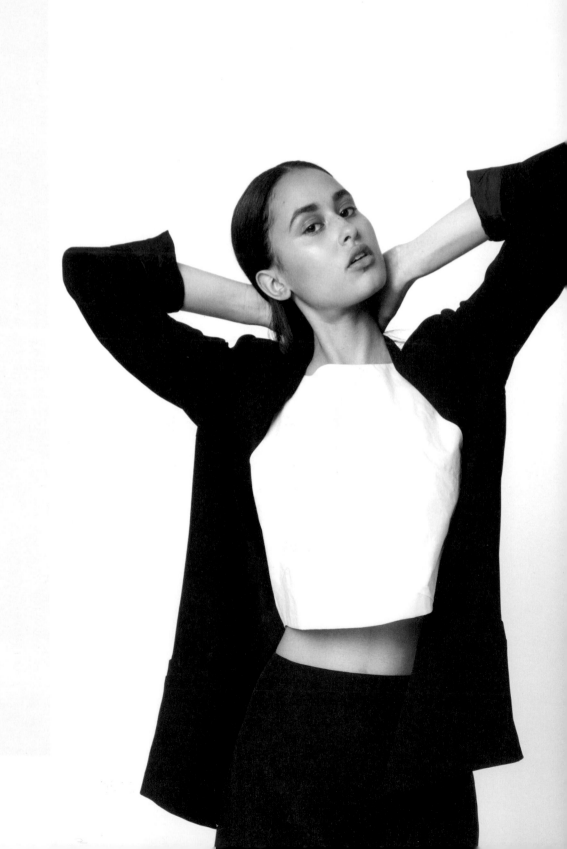

The Curated Closet

A simple system for discovering your personal style and building your dream wardrobe

by Anuschka Rees

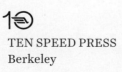

TEN SPEED PRESS
Berkeley

Contents

PART III: BUILD YOUR DREAM WARDROBE

PART IV: THE ART OF SHOPPING

"Buy less,
choose well,
and make
it last."

—*Vivienne Westwood*

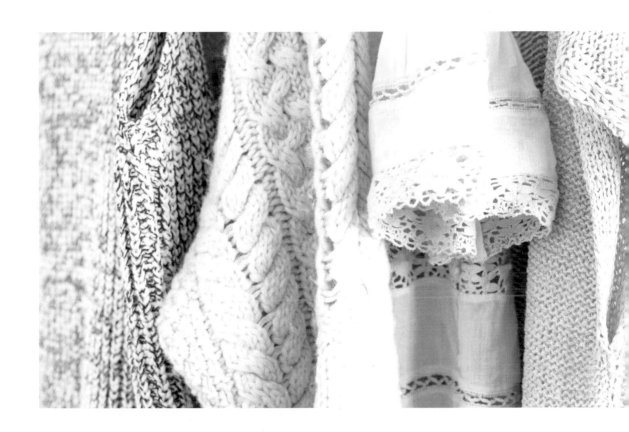

WHAT IS THE CURATED CLOSET?

The Curated Closet is a wardrobe that's perfectly tailored to your unique personal style and your life. It contains everything you need to feel confident and inspired everyday—no more and no less. It is not based on trends, style typologies, or a cookie-cutter list of "wardrobe essentials."

Your life isn't cookie-cutter, so why should your closet be?

Introduction

A tale of bargains, impulse buys, and seasonal must-haves

Here's where it all started: in London, in a studio apartment in Camden town.

That apartment was truly tiny, but the closet inside was huge and jam-packed. I had a ton of clothes—and absolutely nothing to wear.

The strange thing was that, given the time, energy, and money I had spent on my clothes, you'd think I'd have a lot more to show for it. I have always been really into fashion, had a subscription to at least five different fashion magazines from age fifteen onward, and knew my herringbone from my houndstooth early on. I went shopping almost every weekend and spent many evenings on the couch clicking through eBay listings and checking the new arrivals page of my favorite online stores.

In short: I was really excited about fashion and definitely not a newbie. And yet, despite my clear obsession and a full closet, it routinely took me more than an hour to come up with a single outfit to wear to a party, let alone brunch on Sundays or any other occasion that called for more than my go-to jeans and a T-shirt.

Of course, in retrospect, the reasons for my wardrobe troubles now seem pretty obvious.

For starters, I was a poor student living in London, one of the most expensive cities in the world, and, like most other fashion-conscious students on a budget, I tried to make the most of what little money I had by spreading it across as many pieces as possible. I shopped exclusively at fast-fashion, low-priced retailers, kept close tabs on the sales sections at all times, and considered a T-shirt costing more than ten pounds (about fifteen U.S. dollars) a "total rip-off." I was also a complete sucker for great deals like three-for-two, had at least ten different store cards, and would often get up in the middle of the night to stalk whatever "bargain" I had found on eBay.

Ironically, I was pursuing my master's in psychology at that time and really should have known better than to fall for the most basic sales technique there is: short-term price reductions. The fact that for most people all reasonable decision making goes out the window as soon as they are faced with huge price reductions is something you learn in Social Psychology 101. If I saw something on sale that looked interesting, I would rationalize even obvious faults with the piece and lower my standards. I felt that 20 percent off meant I could compromise on things like fit or how the fabric felt on my skin, and of course those were always the pieces that got tossed to the back of my closet after one wear.

Apart from my questionable shopping strategy, I also had a very warped idea of what it meant to dress well. To me, having great style and dressing according to the latest trends were one and the same. And consequently, I also thought there was only one version of style, only one way to dress well that I somehow had to get behind and emulate.

In some ways this idea made things seem relatively straightforward, because it meant there are clear-cut rules and principles that would eventually turn you into the ultrastylish, confident person you long to be, as long as you followed them. And so that's what I tried to do. I studied fashion magazines and runway shows and then tried to hunt down as many budget-friendly alternatives to the season's must-haves as possible. I had my seasonal color type all figured out, was really into body-shape typologies, and filled out every style quiz I could find. I tried to stick exclusively to the recommended colors and silhouettes for my coloring and body type and went on to stock my closet with a crisp white button-down shirt, a black blazer, classic pumps, and all the other pieces that fashion magazines had identified as "essential."

I bought right into the one-size-fits-all mentality that the entire fashion industry so often conveys, perhaps not out of bad will, but for simplicity's sake and to satisfy a demand for quick fixes.

In retrospect, it's no wonder that I was unhappy with my wardrobe. I was stuck in the typical life cycle of the fast shopper.

Because I was all about getting a good deal, I based my purchasing decisions above all on the price of a piece, rather than its quality, how well it fit into my existing wardrobe, or even how much I liked it. I never took the time to truly figure out how I wanted to dress and what type of clothes would work for my life. I didn't have a strategy. I bought clothes on impulse and often based on other people's opinion of them, without listening to my own creative impulses. The combination of all these factors left me with a mishmash of no-good pieces that suited neither my style nor my life. I might have had a full closet, but I didn't have anything to wear that I was actually excited about, and because of that, I always needed more. I kept on buying, more and more of the same low-quality stuff, usually for every new party or event that came up. But every new purchase of course just added to what was already an incoherent mess. Everything was just another quick fix.

Fast forward a couple of years: I still love fashion and still have my magazine subscriptions, but I've stopped chasing trends and wasting my money on flimsy polyester pieces and "seasonal must-haves." I've learned how to buy less but choose better. I own fewer clothes now, but I actually have something to wear.

So what happened? Well, I eventually become so unhappy with the state of my wardrobe that I realized my entire approach needed a serious overhaul. Spending all that money on things I'd never end up wearing started to feel wrong. And then I had a lightbulb moment:

The people I most admire for their style aren't those that follow every trend and dress in designer clothes from head to toe, but people like Sofia Coppola, Charlotte Gainsbourg, and Grace Coddington. These women are style icons not because they follow rules but because they make their own, and each have a strong sense of style and a clear signature look.

After that realization, I set myself a new goal. I wanted to cultivate my own personal style and sort out the mess that was my wardrobe. And on top of that I also wanted to see if there was somehow a system to all of this. Something that other women could replicate, women like me who were into fashion but for whom the traditional "more is more" approach hadn't worked out. And so I started my research. I read and reread every book I could find that was somehow related to fashion and tried out every tip I found in magazines, on myself and every willing friend and family member. I started a blog to write about my favorite techniques and continued to tweak and polish them based on the feedback I got from women of all ages from around the world.

This book is the culmination of all my research. Think of it as a toolbox full of tips, techniques, exercises, and prompts designed to help you cultivate a strong personal style and build a functional wardrobe that allows you to express it.

The perfect wardrobe isn't something that you can cook up in a weekend. Your personal style is the result of many different influences, all the people you have met over the years, all the places you have traveled. It's a truly personal thing that can take a little digging to fully uncover. But don't worry: the process is a lot of fun too!

Plus, once you have cultivated a strong sense of style, become your own best stylist, and built a great wardrobe, those things will stay with you for the rest of your life. And if your wardrobe is important to you and you want to use clothes as a means for self-expression, those are pretty invaluable life skills to have, if you ask me.

Closet Diagnostics

Why you don't have anything to wear

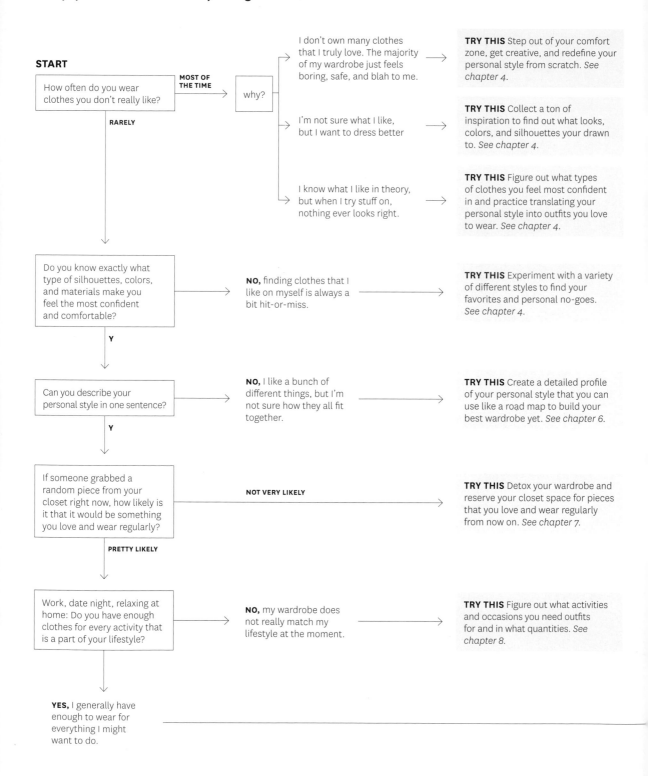

START

How often do you wear clothes you don't really like?

MOST OF THE TIME → why? →

- I don't own many clothes that I truly love. The majority of my wardrobe just feels boring, safe, and blah to me.
  → **TRY THIS** Step out of your comfort zone, get creative, and redefine your personal style from scratch. *See chapter 4.*

- I'm not sure what I like, but I want to dress better
  → **TRY THIS** Collect a ton of inspiration to find out what looks, colors, and silhouettes your drawn to. *See chapter 4.*

- I know what I like in theory, but when I try stuff on, nothing ever looks right.
  → **TRY THIS** Figure out what types of clothes you feel most confident in and practice translating your personal style into outfits you love to wear. *See chapter 4.*

RARELY ↓

Do you know exactly what type of silhouettes, colors, and materials make you feel the most confident and comfortable?

→ **NO,** finding clothes that I like on myself is always a bit hit-or-miss.
→ **TRY THIS** Experiment with a variety of different styles to find your favorites and personal no-goes. *See chapter 4.*

Y ↓

Can you describe your personal style in one sentence?

→ **NO,** I like a bunch of different things, but I'm not sure how they all fit together.
→ **TRY THIS** Create a detailed profile of your personal style that you can use like a road map to build your best wardrobe yet. *See chapter 6.*

Y ↓

If someone grabbed a random piece from your closet right now, how likely is it that it would be something you love and wear regularly?

→ **NOT VERY LIKELY**
→ **TRY THIS** Detox your wardrobe and reserve your closet space for pieces that you love and wear regularly from now on. *See chapter 7.*

PRETTY LIKELY ↓

Work, date night, relaxing at home: Do you have enough clothes for every activity that is a part of your lifestyle?

→ **NO,** my wardrobe does not really match my lifestyle at the moment.
→ **TRY THIS** Figure out what activities and occasions you need outfits for and in what quantities. *See chapter 8.*

↓

YES, I generally have enough to wear for everything I might want to do.

NO, I don't really have a problem with overspending or impulse shopping. → Your closet is in good shape. Lucky you! Use this book to refine your personal style and perfect your wardrobe.

Do you have a tendency to spend over your budget or shop on impulse? Can you simply not help yourself when you see an irresistible bargain, deal, or sale?

YES, that sounds like me. → **TRY THIS** Identify your personal triggers for overspending and rethink your budgeting strategy. *See chapter 18.*

MAKE THE RIGHT DECISIONS

What's your success rate when it comes to making smart purchasing decisions? Do you love and wear most of the clothes you buy for a long time? Or do a lot of them end up at the back of your closet with the tag still on?

DON'T MAKE THE RIGHT DECISIONS

Much of what I buy turns out to be less useful than I thought. → **TRY THIS** Up your success rate by using a clear decision-making process to recognize no-good pieces before you buy. *See chapter 17.*

N

Do you feel as if your outfits often don't look as good as they do on other people? Are they missing that special something?

YES, my styling skills could use some brushing up. → **TRY THIS** Experiment! Figure out how to make the most of every piece in your wardrobe and build up a repertoire of styling tricks. *See chapter 15.*

Y

Do you find it easy to mix and match the pieces in your wardrobe into lots of different combinations? Or do most of your clothes work only as part of a few different outfits?

NO, many of my clothes don't work that well with each other, so I repeat the same looks over and over again. → **TRY THIS** Build a mixable wardrobe of key pieces, basics, and statement pieces. *See chapter 9.*

PART I

THE BASICS

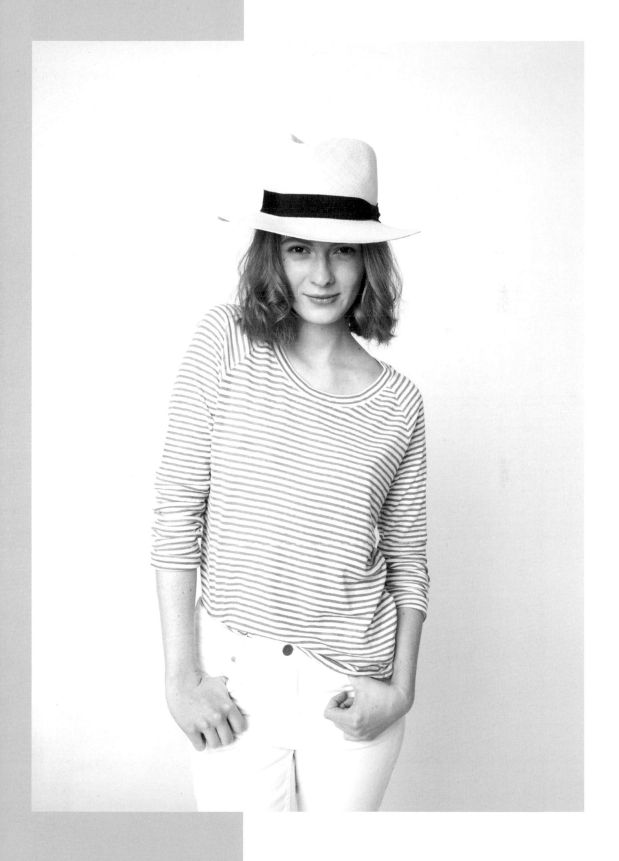

01 / The Curated Closet philosophy

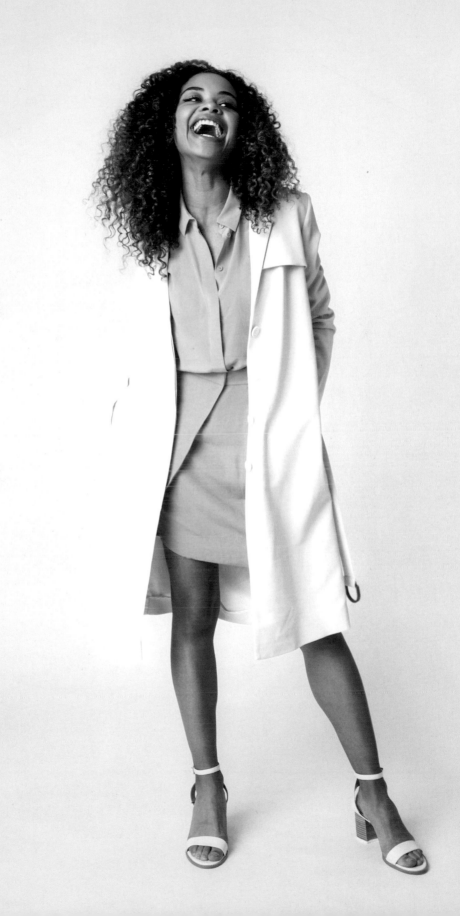

Let's talk strategy! A complete introduction to the five key principles that every single tip, technique, and exercise in this book is based on.

1. Be selective: Reserve your closet space for items you love 100 percent

Training yourself to become more selective is the single most effective thing you can do to upgrade your wardrobe. Try to think of your closet as an exclusive, members-only club. Only pieces that you love and are truly excited to wear get an invite. Anything ill-fitting, scratchy, worn-out, barely "good enough," or that simply doesn't suit your personal style is not invited.

Now, it may seem common sense to not buy things you don't really like all that much, let alone keep them in your closet or even wear them, but, in reality, we often make do with imperfect things:

- We buy items that we only half like because they are on sale or a "good deal."
- We wear clothes that are so uncomfortable we need to take them off as soon as we get home.
- We keep items that stopped fitting years ago just in case they fit again someday.
- We wear shoes that we can hardly walk in and that leave our feet covered in blisters.
- We force ourselves to wear pieces that we feel only so-so about because they were expensive and we don't want to let that "investment" go to waste.
- We wear worn-out, scruffy pieces around the house and hope nobody is going to stop by unannounced.
- We wear clothes that ride up and tug in all the wrong places.
- We wear outfits that don't make us feel confident or inspired because we simply don't have anything better in our wardrobe.

And why do we do all these things? Why do we spend our money on stuff that we don't even like? Why do we put up with clothes that are uncomfortable?

Because it's easier, at least in the short term. It takes less mental energy to just make a quick decision and buy that top you need for an event at work, even when you don't really like how it fits around your bustline, than it is to spend another hour looking for one you really love. It's easier to just keep wearing your worn-out, stretchy pair of jeans than it is to go through the oftentimes exhausting process of finding a pair that fits the individual contours of your body perfectly. Most people are also more comfortable just putting up with battered feet after a night spent in ill-fitting heels than admitting that those eighty dollars were not well spent. In the same way, it's easier to keep telling yourself you'll fit into your old favorites again someday, even though they're now two sizes too small, than it is to let go of them.

Of course, all these decisions make life easier only right in that moment. In the long run, having to keep readjusting a skirt that rides up with each step or deal with straps that painfully dig into your shoulders each time you wear a no-good piece is way more stressful. It's also stressful to have to comb through piles of clothes each morning just to find one acceptable outfit. And of course, if what you wear is important to you, not being able to find anything you truly love will affect your confidence levels eventually, and that's stressful too.

> In the long run, putting more effort into selecting the right piece always pays off.

But because of our natural human tendency to conserve energy in the short term and choose the easiest route when possible, being more selective when it comes to your wardrobe is something you actively have to practice.

As you work through this book, you will come across many different techniques that will not only help you be more selective but also make the process feel easier. You'll learn how to assess the quality of potential new wardrobe

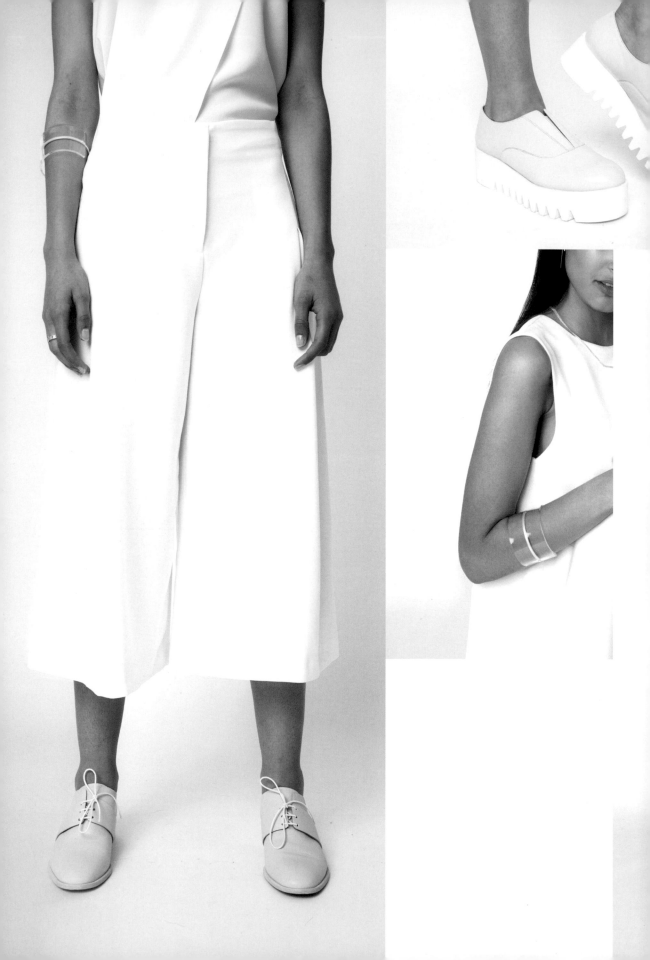

additions and how to recognize pieces that may look great on the hanger but won't feel good on your body by the end of a long day. You'll develop strategies for how to resist clever marketing ploys, de-stress your shopping experience, and prevent impulse buys and other less-than-ideal purchasing decisions. And most important: You will become more and more aware of your own personal style and individual wardrobe needs and eventually be able to tell in an instant whether an item suits your style and works with the rest of your clothes or not.

2. Be authentic: Forget conventional style typologies like "classic" or "bohemian" and create your own unique look

Style typologies and lists of "wardrobe essentials" are to style seekers what fad diets are to people who want to lose a few pounds: quick-fix, one-size-fits-all solutions that make you feel as if you are making progress for a while but ultimately won't help you address the root of the problem.

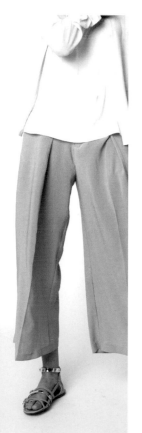

When I was younger and still very unsure about my own style, I took these style typologies very seriously and thought if only I managed to curate every single piece recommended for my "type," I would finally become the stylish and impeccably dressed woman I longed to be. Most quizzes put me in the "classic" category, and so I went on to stock my wardrobe with button-down shirts, ballet flats, and, of course, a trench coat. The first time I wore that trench coat, I felt like a little girl playing dress-up with her mother's wardrobe, but I tried my best to ignore that feeling. I was following the advice of fashion experts after all; surely they knew what they were talking about, and I probably just had to get used to my chic new look.

And that's the problem with style typologies, lists of "wardrobe essentials," and really any fashion advice that tells you what to wear or put in your wardrobe: They present you with a neat little ready-made formula for style and thereby keep you from thinking things through for yourself and following your own creative impulses. They promote the idea that "style" can happen in only one of three to seven ways (depending on how many magazine pages need to be filled) and that dressing well is about how well you stick to those rules.

Fad diets, style typologies, and "wardrobe essentials" lists are popular for the same reason: they satisfy a demand for a quick solution and simplify what can feel like a daunting process down to a set of easy-to-follow rules that seem manageable.

The problem is that a ready-made, one-size-fits-all approach can give you only a ready-made, one-size-fits-all wardrobe. Following rules and blueprints is not going to help you cultivate a strong sense of style, because your personal style is just that: deeply personal. Sure, you may like a lot of the same colors, materials, or cuts as someone else, but the way you combine these into outfits, the pieces you choose for different occasions, and how you style your looks are all a reflection of your unique likes and dislikes and the influences that you have picked up over the years.

> True personal style is always custom-made, so building a cookie-cutter wardrobe makes little sense.

For example, I have a friend who always wears the most amazing flowy dresses paired with long necklaces and a hat. Based on that description, a run-of-the-mill style quiz would probably classify her as the "bohemian" type and recommend she stock her wardrobe with floral pieces, fringed bags, lots of patterns, and warm, bright colors. Her wardrobe in real life? Cool and monochromatic, full of understated accessories, and not a pattern in sight. Her style doesn't fit into any of the traditional style types, and yet it's completely cohesive. Each of her outfits represent her unique aesthetic perfectly. It's impossible to describe her style in a few words, but that doesn't really matter, because once you have found your personal style, it only needs to make sense to you.

Of course, when it comes to building a great wardrobe, personal style is only one part of the puzzle. How you implement that style (in other words, which exact pieces you include as part of your wardrobe) depends on many other factors, including your specific lifestyle, your body, your favorite fits and fabrics, your budget, and even your typical laundry routine. And all these are, again, things that are solely defined by your individual preferences, something to which no ready-made list of "wardrobe essentials" could possibly be tailored.

So, if you have picked up this book expecting a fail-proof wardrobe plan that you can replicate, I have to disappoint you. On no page of this book will I tell you what to wear, which pieces to include in your wardrobe, or what kind of top to match with which kind of bottom. What I will do is show you how you can figure all these things out for yourself, how to discover your unique likes and dislikes, and how to combine everything into a functional personal style that's authentic because it's truly your own.

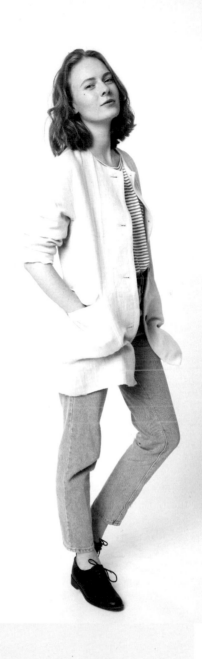

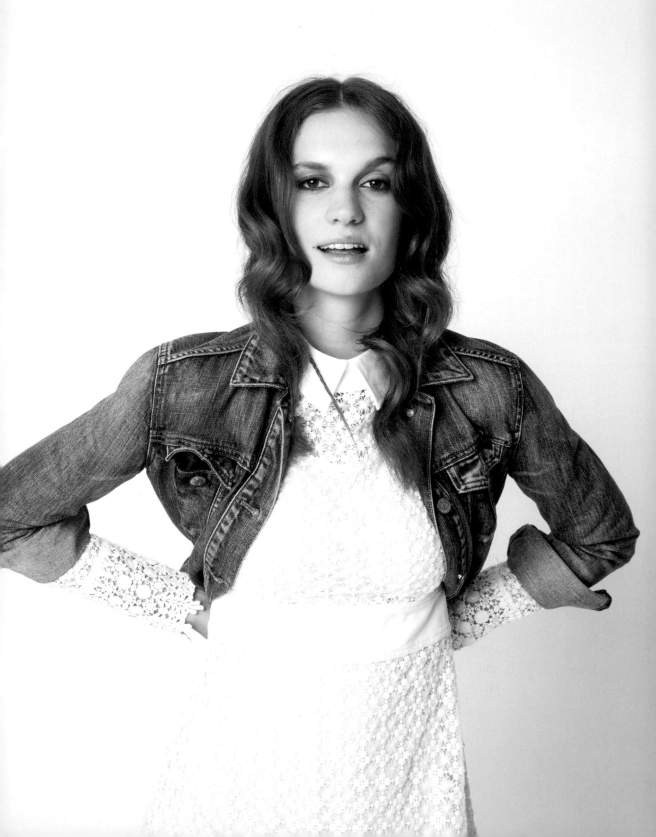

3. Aim for quality: Build a wardrobe of high-quality pieces that last more than just a few years

Only a few years ago, the concept of "quality over quantity" seemed inherently flawed to me. I thought, why in the world would I want to blow all my money on one pair of jeans, when I can have five pairs instead?

I was firmly in the "more is more" camp, and so I put up with shoes that gave me blisters, flimsy polyester T-shirts that felt itchy, and pants that I had to readjust after every tiny movement, all in exchange for having more (equally flawed) options hanging in my closet. I didn't bother caring properly for my clothes or storing them right, and to me, it wasn't a big deal if a garment fell apart in the wash, a seam ripped, or a heel broke off of one of my shoes. Each individual piece simply wasn't worth much to me, not just monetarily but also within the context of my jam-packed wardrobe.

The result of this approach was that I usually threw out the majority of my clothes at the end of a season: some pieces because they had literally fallen apart, others because the fabric was covered in pills, and many because they had simply turned out to be so uncomfortable or ill-fitting, I couldn't bear the thought of ever wearing them again. And so, about twice a year after a thorough clean-out, my closet always looked frighteningly empty to me and the whole vicious cycle started again . . .

Sounds terribly wasteful? It was. Fortunately, my strategy did a complete 180 almost as soon as my goal had shifted from "be fashionable" to "cultivate my own personal style." That process happened quite naturally for me, as it does for most people: once you become more selective about what you keep in your closet, you'll attach a bigger value to each individual piece and will probably no longer be satisfied with cheap, badly manufactured stuff. You'll want clothes that feel good on your skin. Clothes that are sturdy and durable and that won't fall apart after a couple of seasons. Clothes that fit the contours of your body well, without distorting your silhouette or restricting movement.

Aiming for quality goes hand in hand with building a great wardrobe that expresses your style and supports your life. And that's why this book—in addition to making sure your wardrobe aligns with your style from an aesthetic point of view— emphasizes choosing clothes that are high-quality, functional, and made to last.

You'll learn how to put together a wardrobe that works for your lifestyle, is as versatile as possible, and gives you tons of outfit options for all your activities. You'll become a pro at assessing the quality of garments based on factors like the craftsmanship of its seams or the composition of its fabric. You'll get to know your own subjective preferences for materials, silhouettes, and details inside out. There's also a whole chapter dedicated to choosing clothes that fit well, so you'll eventually be able to instantly tell whether the construction of a potential new piece aligns well with the individual proportions of your body.

And don't worry if you are on a budget: you don't need a fat wallet to put together a high-quality wardrobe. The quality of a garment is rarely perfectly correlated with its price, and once you know all about assessing garments, you'll be well equipped to find high-quality pieces at all price points.

4. Style trumps fashion: Get excited about fashion trends that suit your own style, but ignore all others

One of my biggest style-related pet peeves is the idea of "keeping up with fashion."

It suggests that fashion is the equivalent of a law that it is our duty, as respectable people, to uphold. It suggests that the key to dressing well is following the rules and wearing whichever trends and must-haves the fashion world is prescribing that season, regardless of whether we actually like them or not.

Of course, that's a very literal interpretation of the phrase, but it nevertheless captures the underlying message that the fashion industry is sending to women to drive sales, using headlines like "5 Skirts You Need This Spring" or "Essential Trends for This Year." And because of that, most women I know still do feel at least some pressure to dress in line with the trends, worry about certain things looking "outdated," and use current fashion do's and don'ts as the deciding factor when it comes to choosing outfits.

Most women think you have to be fashionable to be well dressed. And that's what I thought too until only a few years ago. But here's what I've learned since:

Being fashionable is totally optional.

Some of the biggest style icons of the last century were people who explicitly did *not* follow every new trend out there and instead had their own very distinctive looks from which they rarely strayed. Think Marlene Dietrich, Grace Jones, or Marilyn Monroe and also modern style icons like Jenna Lyons, Tilda Swinton, or Angelina Jolie. In fact, some of the most consistent style icons of today come from the fashion industry itself, like Karl Lagerfeld, Anna Wintour, and Emmanuelle Alt. All these people are stylish, not despite the fact that they don't follow trends but *because* of it. They know exactly what they like and what they don't like. Their style is iconic because it is completely authentic.

That's not to say I am against fashion, not at all. And having your own personal style and being into fashion aren't mutually exclusive. What's key is that, rather than seeing fashion as a ubiquitous standard, you see it for what it really is: an art form. Like music, architecture, and literature, fashion is a form of art and an important part of human culture that reflects both bigger cultural shifts and smaller movements (such as seasonal trends). Now, what separates fashion from many other art forms is that it is much more prevalent in everyday life. In that sense, it is perhaps most comparable to music, another art form that most people have an opinion about. But unlike with clothes, you wouldn't make yourself listen to songs all day just because they are at the top of the charts right now or because a "hip" person told you to, right? Of course not; you listen to music that you like. And that's exactly what it should be like with fashion as well.

Just like music, fashion should be about celebrating creativity and having fun. You should not feel bad about wearing a supertrendy head-to-toe look if you love it, but you also shouldn't feel bad about wearing something that's not in line with what's currently considered to be *the* look. If you are a creative person, fashion can be a great outlet for experimentation, inspiration, and just having fun. I personally still get just as exited about Fashion Week nowadays as I did during my shopaholic phase. But what's changed is that now, instead of treating all the new trends and pieces like a to-do list, I think of them like a buffet. I'm free to pick and choose. If I see a look and immediately love it, I will look to buy something in that style and continue wearing it long after it's gone out of style again. But if I don't see anything that suits my style, I'll just stick to my old favorites for that season.

In this book, we'll focus on style rather than fashion. Fashion can be fun and inspiring, but it is volatile, and there is no guarantee that the trend you've so madly fallen in love with just a few months ago will still look just as enticing to you once the season is over. If your ultimate goal is to build a great wardrobe that you will love for more than a couple of seasons, your personal style should always be your primary compass.

5. Put in the work: Invest time and thought into developing your style and selecting the perfect garments

Many people have the misconception that a great sense of style is one of these things you either have or don't have. They imagine that people who are well dressed simply get up in the morning and, through some act of divine inspiration, come up with a perfectly original and brilliant new outfit idea.

On the other end of the spectrum, there are the people who believe the exact opposite: they think of clothes and fashion as simple, almost trivial, and something they should be able to master without too much effort. But when things then turn out be a little trickier than expected, they feel as though they've failed, and their wardrobes become huge sources of stress and frustration for them.

So who is right? Neither, because styling is a skill like any other. And that means anyone can learn it and you don't have to be born with a natural talent for it. But you also cannot expect to be great at styling without putting in any effort at all.

Like everything in life, styling takes practice.

It takes time to train your eye, experiment with different aesthetics, and develop a sense of style that feels natural and effortless to you. It takes time to figure out which types of pieces work best for your lifestyle and to curate a versatile wardrobe. And it takes time to then learn how to best utilize those pieces to create outfits that you love.

The bottom line is that if you want great style and a wardrobe that reflects it, you need to put in the work. But the good news is that, no matter what your wardrobe looks like right now, you can get it back in shape and even have fun doing so. You can cultivate a strong personal style, even if right now you have no idea what that could possibly look like. All it takes is a little time, a little effort, and the right techniques.

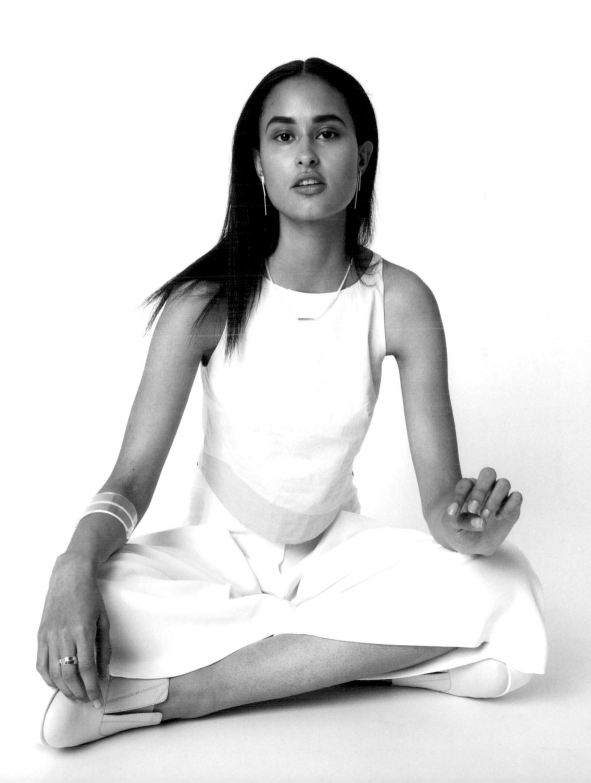

MINIMALISM AND THE CURATED CLOSET

If I had to sum up my wardrobe and my overall approach to clothes in one word, it would be *minimalist*, even though my personal style is not minimalist in an aesthetic sense. And guess what: the tools and techniques in this book will help you build a minimalist wardrobe too! No matter whether your style is stark and minimal or a crazy mix of punk rock and gothic Elizabethan vibes.

Because here's the deal: minimalism as an *aesthetic style* and minimalism as a *lifestyle philosophy* are two very different things.

MINIMALISM AS A STYLE

As a style, the term *minimalist* (or *minimal*) can be used to describe any concept that's pared down to its most essential elements. Some examples:

- Minimal art, which became popular in the 1960s as a counter movement to the bold and colorful abstract expressionism of the post–World War II years, features a much subtler use of color and often a focus on clean geometric shapes.
- In literature, Ernest Hemingway and Samuel Beckett are often cited as great minimalist writers because of their very matter-of-fact way of putting things, without metaphors, flowery descriptions, or adverbs.
- And, of course, minimalism as a visual style also plays a huge role in the fashion world. Calvin Klein, Jil Sander, and Balenciaga are all labels that are popular for their stripped-down aesthetics. Their pieces are usually constructed with a special focus on functionality and a clean, modern silhouette, with minor to no embellishments and a toned-down color palette.

MINIMALISM AS A LIFESTYLE

The key idea of minimalism as a lifestyle philosophy is no different from that of minimalism as a style: remove what's nonessential or what isn't working to put a greater focus on what is left. Or, in other words, get rid of everything that doesn't make you happy or enrich your life to make space for stuff that does.

But there is one big difference: in art, design, and fashion, minimalism is a specific style that can be identified by a set of characteristics, just like many other styles.

But when it comes to minimalist living, there is no one way to do it. Why? Because being a minimalist in itself is not the goal; it's always only a means to an end. And that end is usually less stress and more happiness. Living simply is essentially just a technique that you use to improve your daily life, like yoga, healthy eating, meditation, or whatever else you do to stay happy and sane, and that's why you can pick and choose how and to what extent you want to incorporate aspects of minimalist living into your life.

It's not about owning or doing as little as possible. It's about owning and doing the right things, things that add value to your life.

Minimalism is all about that little bit of extra intention and making conscious choices. It's about being thoughtful and selective and figuring out what's right for you and your life specifically instead of blindly following trends or the advice of other people.

That extra intentionality is what makes my wardrobe minimalist. And it's what this entire book is about: being superclear about how you want to dress, based on your unique personal style and lifestyle, and then putting together a functional wardrobe that contains exactly what you need to express that style.

Minimalism is not a numbers game. So don't worry—I'm not going to ask you to throw out three-quarters of your entire closet or learn how to make do with two pairs of shoes. The goal is not to build a wardrobe that is as small as possible but one that is as functional and personalized as possible. Sure, most people who go through the process, me included, do end up with a somewhat smaller wardrobe, but that is only because once they have figured out how they want to dress, they see no point in holding on to all those imperfect pieces that have accumulated over the years. But it is completely up to you how many clothes you to want to include in your final wardrobe. And that number may shrink and grow over the years as your style continues to evolve.

How to use this book

Are you ready to build your best wardrobe yet? Here's everything you need to know to get started.

No matter whether you are a long-time fashion enthusiast with closet troubles or a total beginner, this book will teach you how to take your closet to the next level, step by step and with a lot of fun and a little self-discovery along the way.

Here is a quick overview of everything you'll learn, do, and discover.

THE CURATED CLOSET SYSTEM

We'll start with a thorough inspection of your current style and closet situation so you'll know exactly what to focus on throughout the next chapters. Perhaps you've already followed the flow chart on pages 6 and 7 to diagnose your closet's weak spots. In the next chapter, you'll find a comprehensive questionnaire (page 33) to help you dig even deeper and analyze your style and wardrobe from all angles. Based on that, you can then put together a little mission statement for your style journey ahead.

DISCOVER YOUR PERSONAL STYLE

In this section, you'll learn how to discover (or refine) your personal style through a series of creative exercises and lots of helpful prompts. You'll immerse yourself in inspiration, try on a ton of clothes, and figure out what colors, cuts, and combinations make you feel inspired and confident. In the last chapter of this section, you'll find out how to create an in-depth profile of your unique personal style. That profile is what you'll use as a road map for the revamping of your closet that we will work through in the rest of the book. So don't skip this one!

BUILD YOUR DREAM WARDROBE

Now comes the nitty-gritty: curating your closet! This section features plenty of tips, step-by-step instructions, and concrete examples to help you put together a versatile, personalized wardrobe that's just right for your style and your life. We'll start with a little prep work: detoxing your closet and analyzing your day-to-day lifestyle.

I'll then show you three different concepts you can use to map out your ideal wardrobe: closet composition, color palettes, and outfit formulas. Use them all together or just pick and choose one or two favorites. And to make sure your ideal wardrobe is well tailored to your professional life, there's also a whole chapter on how to tweak your closet for work (page 148).

Once you know exactly what you want your closet to look like, it's time to turn that dream into a reality. You'll learn how to do just that with the step-by-step guide on page 161. And lastly, you'll get to know your new and improved wardrobe inside out and become your own best stylist.

THE ART OF SHOPPING

This section is packed with lots of practical techniques that you can use to make smarter purchasing decisions as you overhaul your wardrobe and for the rest of your life. Topics include how to become a more selective shopper, find pieces you'll love for seasons to come, and make the most of your budget. There are also two chapters dedicated to garment quality (page 222) and proper fit (page 238) to help you stock your wardrobe with high-quality, great-fitting clothes that make you look and feel great.

And finally, the last chapter in this book is all about maintenance: how to keep your closet in good shape throughout the year (page 248).

HOW TO WORK THROUGH THIS BOOK

It is completely up to you to what extent you use the tools and techniques in this book. If you want to give your closet a serious upgrade, work your way through each section and rebuild your wardrobe step by step. Or, if you are already pretty happy with your closet, feel free to choose your own program of exercises to put the finishing touches on your style or improve individual aspects of your wardrobe.

Whether you decide to complete all the exercises in this book or design your own program, I definitely recommend you *read* through the whole book, because many of the concepts and techniques build upon each other.

HOW LONG WILL IT TAKE ME TO CURATE MY CLOSET?

The answer is, it depends. Some of the exercises might be super simple for you, and you'll be able to whiz through them. Others might be a little tougher, and you'll be scratching your head for a while. If you already feel confident about your style or have experience when it comes to curating your closet, you'll have an easier time with certain techniques and can focus on really defining your unique aesthetic and perfecting your wardrobe. If you are a total newbie and have never given much thought to how you dress, it will probably take you a little longer to complete some of the exercises. But you'll get there, I promise.

And if you are somewhere in the middle, just take it step by step. Spend as much time as you need on each exercise, and don't forget to have fun!

SET UP A STYLE FILE

What's a style file? It's a place where you can collect all your ideas, inspiration material, and answers to the different questions and exercises in this book.

Your style file could be a simple folder on your laptop (or, if you prefer pen and paper, or a box or binder), to house your notes, cutouts, and other bits and pieces that you'll likely accumulate throughout this process.

 To let you know when it's time to add to your style file, every exercise in this book features this little hanger icon to the left.

02/

Getting started: Define the status quo and set style goals

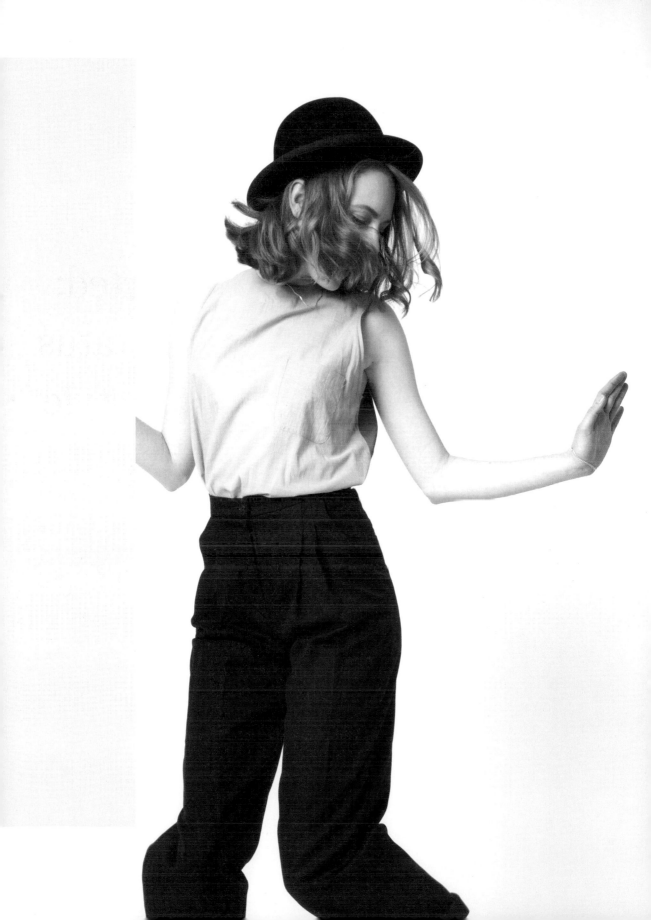

The best place to start your style journey is your current closet. What do you already like about the way you dress, what needs changing, and what skills do you want to learn? That's what we'll figure out in this chapter!

Your very first to-do is an easy one: document your outfits for two weeks. Then crack open your style file, put on your thinking cap, and complete the questionnaire on pages 33 and 34. Try to answer each question in as much detail as possible. Your goal here is to get a complete overview of your current wardrobe and your biggest strengths and weaknesses when it comes to shopping for new piece, styling outfits, and so on.

Let's get started!

Step 1: Document your outfits

When it comes to style, details matter. So, rather than writing a loose recap of your day-to-day outfits, do this: take a quick photo of every single outfit you are wearing for two full weeks and keep a log of the occasions or environments where you wore each outfit. For example: school, client meeting, running errands, and so on. To get the most accurate assessment of how you are currently using your wardrobe, try to pick two regular weeks that are a good representation of your typical lifestyle.

Step 2: Status quo questionnaire

 Once you have documented two weeks' worth of outfits, gather all your pictures in front of you and answer the questions below one by one.

YOUR STYLE

- What was your favorite outfit that you wore during the last two weeks and why? How did that outfit make you feel?
- What was your least favorite outfit and why? How did it make you feel?
- On a scale of 1 to 10, how happy were you overall with your outfits during these past two weeks?
- Describe your current style in three adjectives.
- List your five most-worn colors during the last two weeks. How well do you feel these represent your individual preference for colors?
- What type of silhouettes and fits did you wear most often (for example, skinny jeans, flared skirts, loose tops, fitted blazers)? Why?
- Do you tend to follow a specific formula for putting together your outfits? Do you have a uniform?
- How much variety do you need? Do you enjoy wearing a wide range of different colors, silhouettes, and details, or do you like having a signature look that you repeat with only minor variations?
- Do you prefer being overdressed or underdressed?
- Do you want people to notice your clothes?
- How do you usually style your outfits? Do you often tuck in your tops or roll up your sleeves? What type of accessories do you wear most often?
- Overall, how comfortable were your outfits? What qualities distinguish the most comfortable from the least comfortable pieces in your wardrobe, in terms of fit, material, or details?

- Looking at the pictures of your outfits, how well fitting are your clothes?
- Subconsciously or not, our clothes send a message about who we are, our values and personality. What message does your current look send? What would you like it to send?
- Imagine you had total confidence (and unlimited funds to overhaul your wardrobe). Would you keep wearing the same type of outfits as you do now? If not, what would you change?

YOUR WARDROBE

- How easy is it for you to choose an outfit in the morning?
- What percentage of your closet did you wear during the past two weeks?
- How many different seasons do you have to dress for?
- What type of occasions do you have to dress for?
- How well equipped is your wardrobe for each of these occasions?
- What is your stance on repeating outfits? Are you okay with wearing the same head-to-toe look twice in two weeks? How about individual pieces?
- What is your typical shopping strategy? Do you prefer spending your budget on fewer, more expensive clothes or do you tend to spread it across lots of cheaper items?
- What is your typical decision-making process when it comes to buying clothes? Do you often buy things on a whim, or do you tend to make sure you have compared all your options first?

YOU AND CLOTHES

- What is your main motivation for spending time on your style? Do you use fashion as a creative outlet or an expression of your values and personality? Does dressing well give you confidence?
- Which emotions have the biggest impact on how you dress? Do you dress differently when you are very happy or very sad?
- How much does a lack of confidence prevent you from wearing what you like?
- To what extent is what you wear influenced by the people in your life—that is, your close friends, relatives, acquaintances, and coworkers? Do people you are closer to have a stronger influence, or is it the other way around?

Step 3: Write down your style goals

 Take a moment to reflect on your answers to the questionnaire and then write a little summary about the current status of your style, wardrobe, and your goals:

- What do you like about your style and current wardrobe?
- Which aspects of your style and wardrobe need work?
- What new skills do you want to learn?

Here are some examples of what your summary could look like.

Astrid, 36, Needs a New Wardrobe for Her New Life

My closet was perfect for my style and life two years ago, when I still lived in the city and worked full time. But a lot has happened since then: we've moved to a more rural part of the country (with a much harsher year-round climate), I've started working from home . . . and I've got a baby who takes up most of my time and energy. I still love my old clothes, but they just don't work with my new life anymore.

What do you like about your style and current wardrobe?

I own plenty of nice outfits to wear for fancier occasions, like date nights, parties, and evening functions. I've also got a good selection of work pieces that I still get to wear from time to time for client meetings or conferences.

Which aspects of your style and wardrobe need work?

I don't have any clothes that I can wear during the day and that don't make me feel like a total slob. Most of my old clothes aren't comfortable or practical enough for lugging a baby around all day, plus they are hard to clean. My go-to look has been yoga pants and cardigans for the past few months but, honestly, I hate it.

What new skills do you want to learn?

How to dress in a way that's chic but also practical for my day-to-day life.

Kira, 23, Has Outgrown Her Wardrobe

Answering these questions has made me above all realize that I am at a place in my life where I've just outgrown my wardrobe in its current form. I bought most of my clothes while I was still in college, but now that I'm starting my first real job I want to feel more confident, professional. And I want my clothes to say that about me.

What do you like about your style and current wardrobe?

I do like many pieces on their own and I remember why I bought them originally, but somehow the way I wear them, they make me look young or even childish. I've never been afraid of bright colors and patterns, but I think it's the way I mix pieces. I want to try to find ways to wear colors like bright green but in a more adult way, if that makes sense.

Which aspects of your style and wardrobe need work?

My main problem is that I don't like how many of my outfits make me look younger and not so professional. One factor is that I pretty much own only statement pieces, so I definitely need more basics and sophisticated key pieces to pair with my fun stuff. It's also really hot year-round where I live, and I wear a lot of denim shorts with T-shirts but really want to find a better alternative (maybe a chic maxi skirt worn with a linen top), something I can also wear to the office. I've also noticed that I don't really do anything to my outfits in terms of styling, so they look unfinished sometimes.

Another problem is the way I shop. I buy way too much and often without thinking things through properly. That's how I ended up with all those frilly tops and wild colors.

What new skills do you want to learn?

Learn how to build sharp, sophisticated outfits but with a playful touch.

Get better at styling my outfits.

Curb impulse shopping and start planning out my wardrobe as a whole.

Sarah, 28, Is Playing It Too Safe

Compared to my friends, I feel chronically underdressed and just bland, boring, and safe. I used to think that's because I am just not a natural in that area and not particularly interested in fashion anyway, but actually, that's a total lie. I am interested in fashion. I am a very visual, creative person and love reading fashion blogs and studying other people's outfits. I just haven't really spent much thought on my own clothes in recent years, but that's something I want to change now.

What do you like about your style and current wardrobe?

I like the colors in my wardrobe, or rather, the lack thereof. My favorite outfits during the two weeks were anything with my leather jacket and biker boots, and that's the general direction I think I would like to head in stylewise. Apart from that I also preferred all outfits in which I am wearing skinny jeans. I used to think wearing skirts is a good way to hide my thighs, but actually they look fine in jeans, and A-line skirts just aren't really my style.

Which aspects of your style and wardrobe need work?

Pretty much every aspect, except for the colors. The majority of my wardrobe are basic tops, jeans, and plain dark-gray or black skirts. I would love to play around with silhouettes a bit more and just in general add more oomph to everything. I don't want to dress "loud," because that's not my thing, but I just want to have more fun with my clothes. I don't yet know how or in what way, but I would love to have a very clear "look" that people immediately associate with me.

What new skills do you want to learn?

So many! I think I already have good taste when it comes to choosing pieces but I'm not brave enough and tend to go for the safe option. I need to figure out what my personal style is and then learn what type of pieces I can use to create that style.

PART II

DISCOVER YOUR PERSONAL STYLE

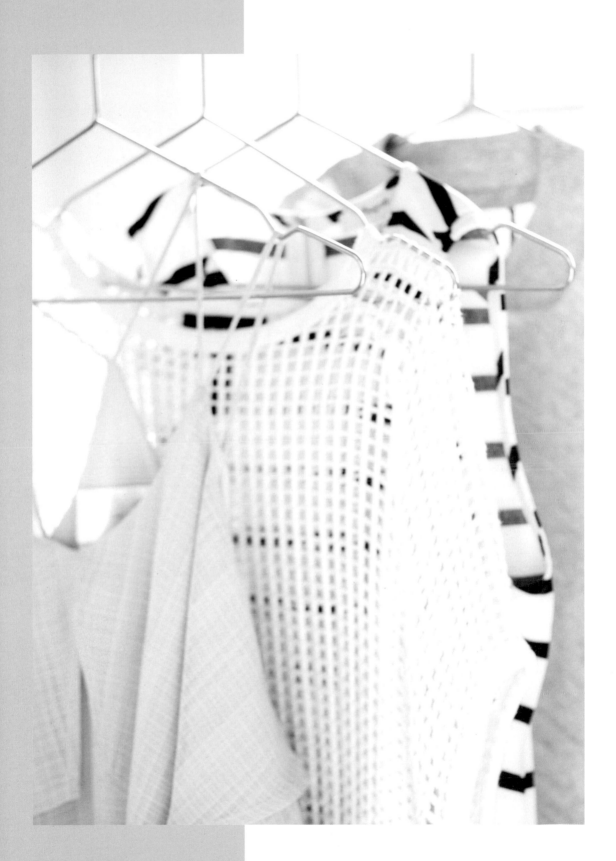

03 / What your clothes say about you

Here's a little food for thought about the role our fashion choices play in our everyday lives. Plus: Learn the secret behind great personal style.

Here's a fun fact for you: the average American spends more than 1,100 dollars on clothes each year and buys close to seventy new pieces. Now, before you start tallying up your last purchases to see how your own spending measures up, let's take a step back.

Why do we care about our clothes at all? Why don't we all just wear an old, comfy sweatshirt and baggy pants and be done with it? Why does style play such an essential role in the lives of so many people? And while we are at it, what exactly is *personal style* anyway?

Behind the clothes

Many people love fashion simply because it's a fun, creative outlet. It's a chance to experiment with colors, shapes, and textures, as an artist would. But there's also a deeper side to it. Because whether or not you are into fashion, your clothes say something . . .

Our clothes tell a story. Our clothes reflect our personality and what's important to us.

The dress you wore that day you met your boyfriend, the oversize sweater you love curling up in on cold nights, the ragged pair of denim shorts you wore almost every day when you backpacked through Europe: your wardrobe is a mix of memories, old and new dreams, and a snapshot of your current state of mind. It's also a toolbox. Because your clothes aren't just mirrors of yourself, they also have the power to transform: the sleek black blazer that you put on

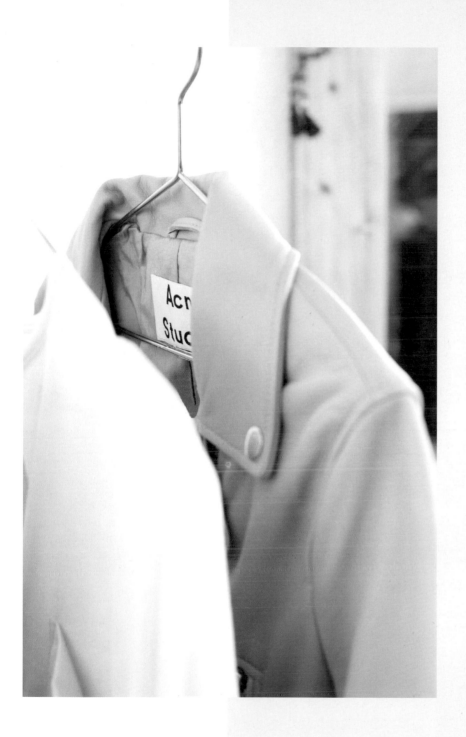

whenever you want to feel extra confident at work; the vintage floral skirt that's so bright and chirpy it always cheers you up; or your most precious pair of earrings that makes every special occasion feel even more special.

Of course, that power can also affect you negatively: If you always reach for dark, shapeless clothes to "hide" from the world when you are having a bad day, you are attaching a negative connotation to that type of outfit. And so, instead of making you feel better, your baggy sweats reinforce your bad emotions because you are literally wearing them around all day.

Clothes can also bring you down when they don't make you feel like *yourself*. If you have ever had to wear a uniform for work or school, you'll know that having to wear clothes you would never in a million years choose to wear yourself can feel strange, uncomfortable even. And that's because you know that clothes always make a statement. We all use what's on the *outside* to make judgments about what's on the *inside*, subconsciously or not. And we know other people judge us the same way.

Having to wear clothes that don't match our inner selves creates cognitive dissonance, and we feel uncomfortable and "dressed up," even when there's nothing wrong with the clothes themselves.

> To be comfortable and confident, we need clothes
> that feel like *us*.

It's like staying at a friend's house or a hotel. You're able to appreciate it, but it just doesn't quite feel like home, where you are surrounded by memories and things you love and that each reflect some small part of you.

If you are not happy with the clothes in your wardrobe at the moment, chances are it's because they don't line up with your personal style just yet. But don't worry: that's something we'll change within the course of this book!

Where personal style comes from

Your style is a mix of preferences for different elements—like colors, silhouettes, textures, and patterns—that all together create a single visual narrative. Your style isn't random and it's also not something you were born with—it's a reflection of your experiences and the associations you picked up over the years.

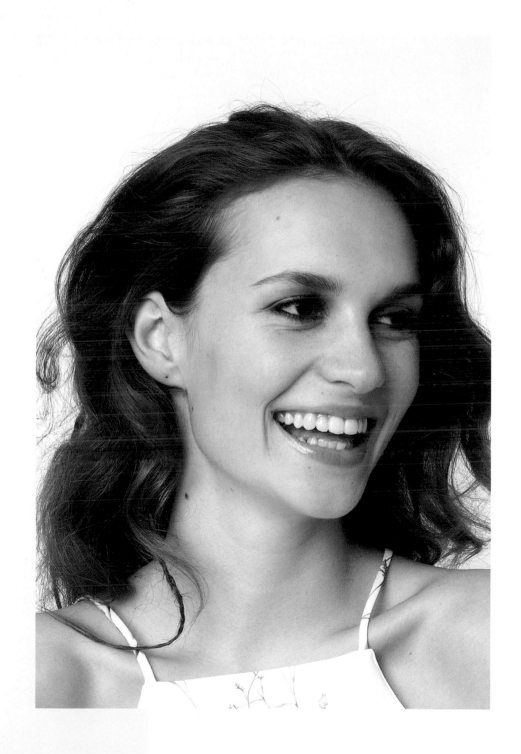

Perhaps at one point you watched a movie, fell in love with its heroine, her confidence and fearlessness, and her go-to look of shift dresses, diamonds, and killer heels. Or perhaps you went through a seventies rock music phase a while back and now associate sequinned tunic dresses and leather jackets with a cool, free-spirited attitude. Or maybe your favorite aunt gave you a pretty turquoise dress for your fifth birthday, and you've loved that color ever since. You have probably forgotten why by now though. Associations like these happen subconsciously for the most part, and that's why they are tricky to trace back. All you know is that you love all things turquoise.

Chapter 21 of this book is all about how to regularly update your wardrobe and keep it tailored to your evolving sense of style.

All great artists have a personal style from filmmakers like Sofia Coppola or Quentin Tarantino to artists like Andy Warhol or Annie Leibovitz to fashion designers like Alexander Wang or Vivienne Westwood. Their styles run as common threads through their entire bodies of work.

Take Sofia Coppola for example. Whether her movies are about an aging movie star, a young queen in the eighteenth century, or celebrity-obsessed teenagers, they all share a sense of melancholy; dreamy, pastel settings; and close-up shots and slow camera pans.

And Annie Leibovitz has photographed hundreds of celebrities since the 1970s. But she always stayed true to her signature style of high contrast, bright lighting, and interesting, often tongue-in-cheek poses.

Sofia Coppola and Annie Leibovitz figured out what they like and they are sticking with it. And you can do the same.

That's not to say personal style can't evolve.

As you go through life, you collect new experiences; you read, watch movies, and discover new things. Your values may change, and so may your lifestyle. You continuously build new associations that blend in with your existing associations to create something new and different over time. One winter you may be super into chunky knit sweaters, wide-leg pants, and ankle boots; the next winter you may prefer a more slim-fitting silhouette and skirts. But once you have truly discovered what you like and what you don't like, that deep underlying preference for a certain aesthetic is likely going to remain stable for a while, and it will be the baseline for all your future style shifts.

How to develop great personal style

Developing a personal style is like creating a sculpture.

Your favorite colors, materials, silhouettes, and other aesthetic preferences are the clay. Before you can do anything else, you first have to gather your clay: dig deep, immerse yourself in inspiration, and experiment with different colors, materials, and silhouettes to find out what you are drawn to. Then start sculpting: figure out how all your different preferences could fit together to create a single visual narrative.

Both of these steps take effort. Artists spend years defining their signature aesthetic. And the same goes for regular people who dress well. They didn't just wake up one morning with a great sense of style; no, they spent years experimenting with different looks, sampled their fair share of now-cringe-worthy outfits, practiced, and fine-tuned.

> Consider these next few chapters your shortcut to great personal style.

If you already have a pretty good idea about how you like to dress, by the end of this section, you'll have a superclear road map of your unique sense of style that you can then use to upgrade your wardrobe.

If you are a complete fashion newbie, get ready to gather your clay and discover what type of clothes make you feel your best.

04 /

Discover your style, phase I: Get inspired

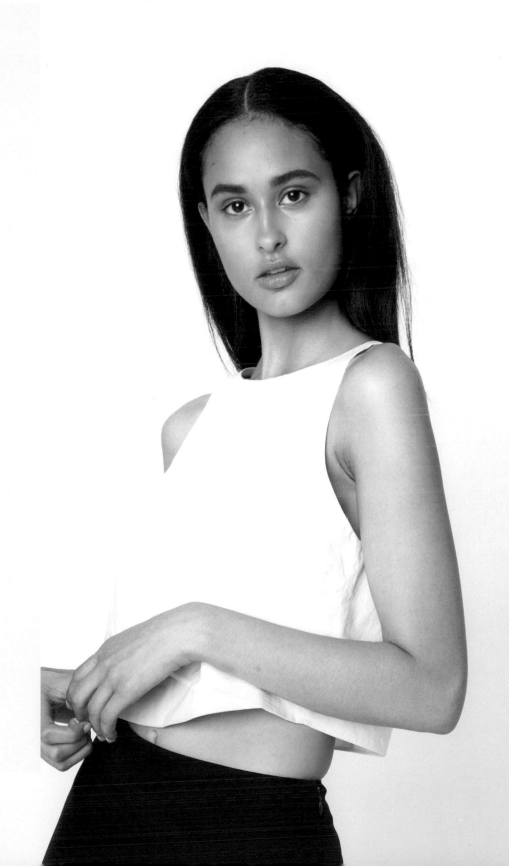

Start honing in on your unique personal style by collecting buckets full of inspiration to discover the aesthetics, colors, and silhouettes that naturally appeal to you.

Collecting inspiration is step 1 of any creative process. The first thing a graphic designer does when creating a logo is to put together an inspiration board that captures the overall vibe of the design she has in mind. Costume designers who are in charge of creating entire wardrobes for characters in movies will spend weeks gathering inspiration from other movies, TV shows, and fashion editorials before they even touch their sewing machine. And the very first step to developing great style is collecting inspiration. You need to see what's out there and expose yourself to as many different styles and aesthetics to see what resonates with you. This chapter will help you do just that.

 Reserve an afternoon or evening to go through blogs, magazines, and other sources and cut out, pin, or save every image that speaks to you in some way in regard to your style. Take notes in your style file along the way.

How to make the most of your inspiration search

SAVE EVERYTHING IN ONE PLACE

Your goal is to end up with a big set of images that you can play around with and organize to spot patterns. The easiest way to store all these images is in a simple folder on your computer. Pinterest boards are great for finding and saving photos, but since you can't easily move them around on a board, I recommend you move them offline into a folder after your initial inspiration search.

Make sure you include in that folder a visual representation of every single thing that inspires you from images you find online to interesting outfit ideas you see on the street. If you don't have a digital image, find one by searching for that item, combination, or outfit directly on Google or Pinterest. Scan pages of magazines and books or just snap a quick picture on your phone.

LOOK FOR THINGS YOU WOULD WEAR IN REAL LIFE

Instead of pinning lots of pretty high-fashion pics, keep your focus on things that will help you build a wardrobe that is right for your current lifestyle. Before you add something to your inspiration folder, ask yourself, would I actually wear this in real life or do I just like this on an abstract level? That's not to say there's no point in looking through fashion editorials at all, because they may still help point you toward certain elements, like specific colors, that you could incorporate into your wardrobe. The trick is to just be aware of this. Feel free to include a gorgeous *Vogue* editorial of models in a dreamy forest scene in your folder if you know that it's the earthy colors of the clothes that inspire you.

DEEPEN YOUR SEARCH

The best inspiration search is both broad and deep: your goal is to expose yourself to as many different aesthetics as possible, to get a feeling for what you are drawn to. But as soon as you have found something you love—for example, a specific piece or a color combination—make sure you go deeper. Search for different ways to wear it, what other people pair with it, and how they style it. If you love an outfit that a blogger is wearing, go through the archives of her blog to see her other looks. In short: Allow yourself to go down rabbit holes.

DELETE IMAGES

Throughout your inspiration search, you'll notice that your likes will become more and more specific. Some images that you liked in the beginning of your search may start to look less appealing to you as you go along. That is a good thing because it means you're starting to develop your own aesthetic. The act of deleting those images is just as important to the style-finding process as finding new images because it helps you set the boundaries for your personal style and define it. So, as soon as you see an image that doesn't look all that great to you anymore, just delete it. Pictures you feel only "meh" about not only distract from others that you love but also skew the overall feel of your collection.

Where to find inspiration

BLOGS AND ONLINE MAGAZINES

Personal style blogs, street style blogs, and online fashion magazines are all great sources for style inspiration. Online fashion magazines and well-known street-style blogs tend to have a strong focus on current fashion trends, so concentrate on personal style blogs if your own preferences don't align well with today's trends. Once you've gone through your go-to sites, Google is your best friend.

Here's how to digitize offline inspiration from books or magazines: (1) take a picture with your phone, (2) scan the page, or (3) search for an image of the item or outfit online.

PRINT MAGAZINES AND FASHION BOOKS

While blogs are a great source for wearable looks, print magazines often offer a different, more refined perspective of fashion with gorgeous editorials and well-thought-out shopping features. Start with your favorite fashion magazines, but make sure you also branch out! And, if you really want to delve deep, check out some books on fashion design, fashion history, or fashion photography.

MOVIES AND TV SHOWS

TV shows and movies, especially those set in current times, are one of my favorite sources for real-life style inspiration because you actually get to see complete wardrobes. Unlike magazines or brand lookbooks, characters in TV shows and movies dress for all sorts of occasions (not just swanky parties) like around the house, at work, and lazy Sundays.

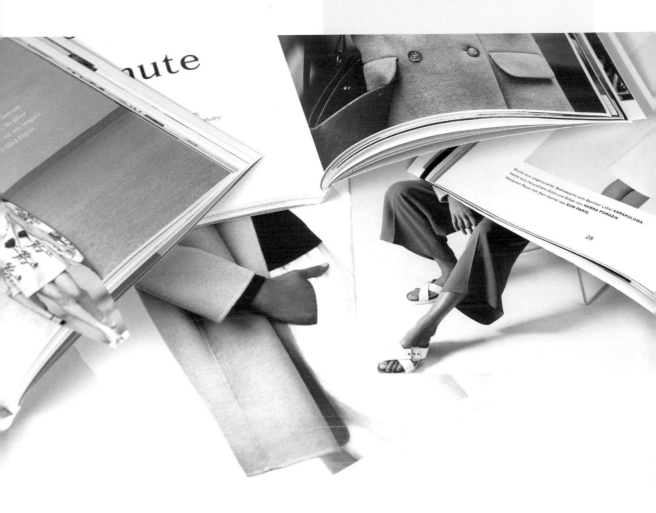

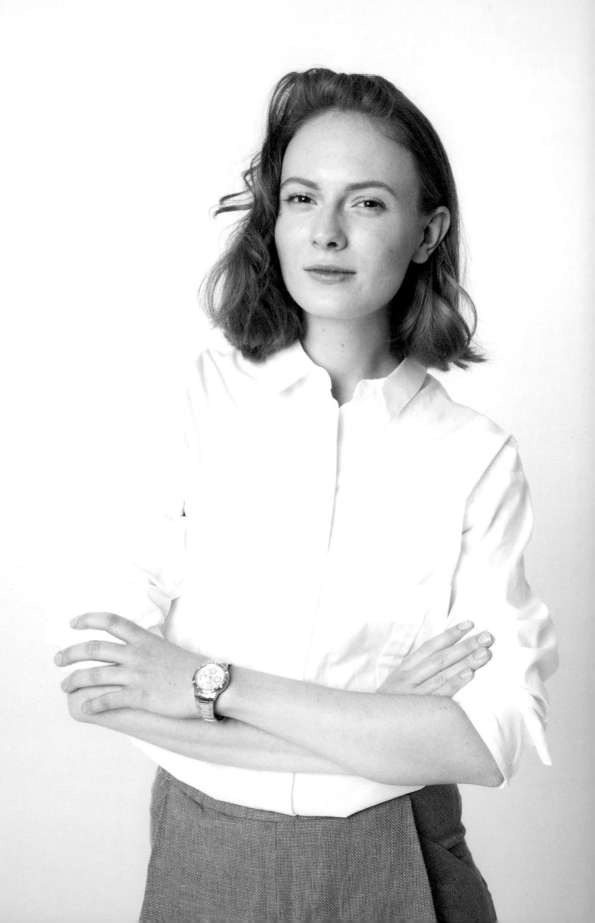

PINTEREST

Pinterest is not only a honeypot for new ideas, but also can be a hugely helpful tool for deepening your search. And that is because Pinterest is basically one huge collection of interconnected inspiration boards of other people. If you find a look that you love, chances are you'll find lots more like it on the board to which it belongs. Another thing about Pinterest that is super convenient is the "Related Pins" feature: if you scroll to the bottom of a pin's page, you'll find lots more similar images.

ONLINE SHOPS, LOOKBOOKS, AND CATALOGUES

Online shops, lookbooks, and other image material from individual brands can be a good source of inspiration, if you love the style of a particular brand. Usually the images from lookbooks and online shops are more stripped down and wearable to showcase the pieces, so if you prefer a simpler look, that's great. Keep in mind that designers will usually style their items in a way that's in line with the overall look of their brand, but that doesn't mean it's the only way to wear them. Do a direct search for specific items to find alternative styling ideas.

PEOPLE WATCHING

Blogs, magazines, and Pinterest aren't the only places to find examples of good personal style. Great style is all around you, so start paying attention and train yourself to become an expert observer! For example, what are people wearing, what colors do they mix, and how do they accessorize their outfits? Take notes about everything that catches your eye and make sure you find representations of it, once you are back home, to add to your set of images.

Where to pay close attention

THE OVERALL VIBE OF THE OUTFIT

Sometimes it's not the individual pieces that draw us to an outfit, but its overall feeling. You may fall in love with an image because of its all-around seventies vibe, edgy punk rock look, or ethereal romantic feeling. Recognizing which overall themes resonate with you may not directly point you toward specific items to include in your wardrobe, but it will definitely help you find your unique aesthetic.

INDIVIDUAL ITEMS

Suede desert boots, a structured panel top, a chic leather jacket paired with a striped, fitted dress: Take note of any individual items or combinations of items in which you could see yourself.

COLORS

Your individual color preferences are a key component of your personal style. As you browse through your inspiration material, pay attention to what kinds of colors you are drawn to and, just as important, which put you off an outfit that you might have otherwise liked.

SILHOUETTES

Keep an eye on what kinds of silhouettes resonate with you, as well as the cut and fit of individual pieces. Do you love high-waisted skirts that are fitted up top but flare out? Are you a fan of skinny jeans with loose-fitting tops? Where do you like skirts and dresses to hit the leg? What type of necklines do you prefer? When it comes to the silhouette of an outfit, an extra inch of length or circumference can make all the difference, so try to be as precise as possible here.

MATERIALS

Look for materials, fabrics, and textures: anything from soft cotton to leather, chunky knitting, or a lightweight chiffon fabric. The material of an item may not always be easy to spot from an image, but if it is clearly visible and essential to the overall look of the piece, make sure you take note.

STYLING

Building a chic outfit is not just about what you wear, but also *how* you wear it. A couple of clever styling techniques can transform even the plainest old-T-shirt-and-jeans combo into a great look. So as you look for inspiration, make sure you also pay attention to all those little details, like how that blogger tucks in her shirt, how she accessorizes her maxi dress, or what makeup she wears with an all-black outfit.

"Help! I Like Styles That Don't Work for My Body Shape."

A common question I get from my readers is this: "What if I am collecting inspiration and repeatedly find myself drawn to things that aren't recommended for my body shape or coloring? Should I just ignore these altogether?"

In short, no!

Here's the thing: in recent years we have all been so inundated with typology-based advice, from various body-shape theories to super in-depth color analysis quizzes, that the idea that only a small set of clothes and colors works for each person has become widely accepted. And that's pretty sad. Sure, there may be a handful of colors in which each one of us looks a little more tired and a few in which we look a little better, but the vast majority of shades will look just fine. The same goes for shapes and silhouettes: yes, a few extreme cuts may make you look a little more bottom-heavy or perhaps a few pounds lighter, but your body is what it is and clothes won't magically change that.

If something is your style and you love it, I believe you should wear it, regardless of whether it supposedly "flatters" your body or doesn't. Plus, if we are being honest, *to flatter* almost always means "makes you look thinner," and that definitely shouldn't be your prime objective when it comes to getting dressed.

If you must, you can always go for a compromise. For example, if you think very loose-fitting boyfriend jeans make you look big, choose a slightly more fitted version. Instead of a bright orange, pick a softer peach, and so on. If it really is something you love, there'll be a way to make it work for your body. And you'll figure out *how* in the next chapter.

But for now, just save every single image that inspires you, even if you're not sure how that particular piece, cut, or color will look on you.

What to do with your inspiration material

Okay, so you've spent at least a full afternoon or evening immersing yourself in inspiration and are now left with a hefty stack of images, online or offline. What now? There are two things: cull and identify patterns.

CULL

Do a quick edit of your entire set of images and weed out anything that doesn't look as appealing anymore or seems redundant. You should also be able to remember exactly what about an image you love and that inspires you in regard to your style. If you can't pinpoint what inspires you in a particular image, toss it.

IDENTIFY PATTERNS

 This last step is where the real magic happens. Look at your entire selection of images from a bird's-eye perspective and break it down into concrete themes and elements.

To get started, choose one of the categories from pages 55–56, such as colors and then write down any individual shades or color combinations that stand out from your set of images. Next, look for individual pieces, silhouettes, styling techniques, and so on. Don't worry about analyzing every tiny aspect of an image; just focus on the dominant patterns and qualities that you found yourself drawn to over and over again, because these are what will likely represent the essence of your style.

In the end, you should be left with a tidy list of elements that you love and might want to include in your wardrobe. Think of that list as a preliminary recipe for your ideal style, a first draft. In the next step, you'll get a chance to test-drive and fine-tune it. Here's an example of what your list may look like:

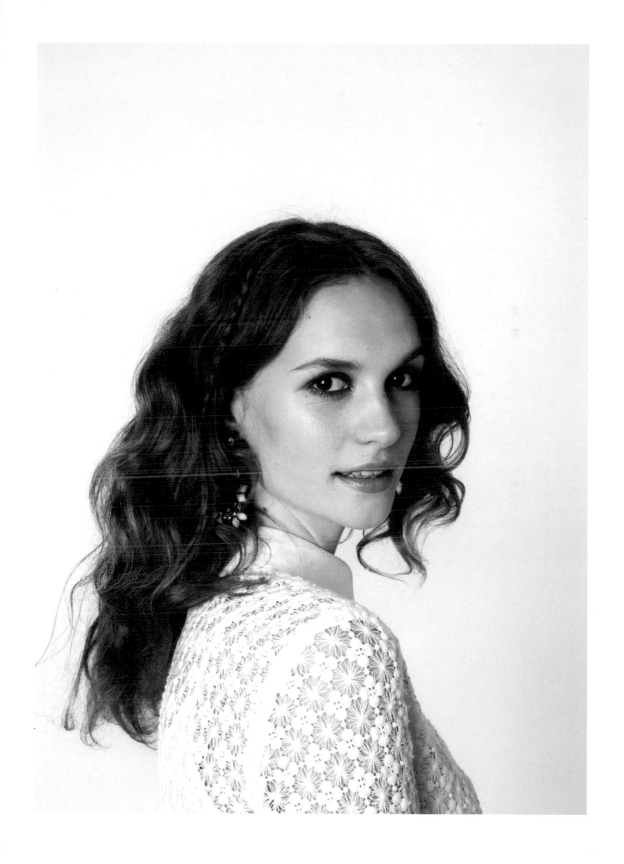

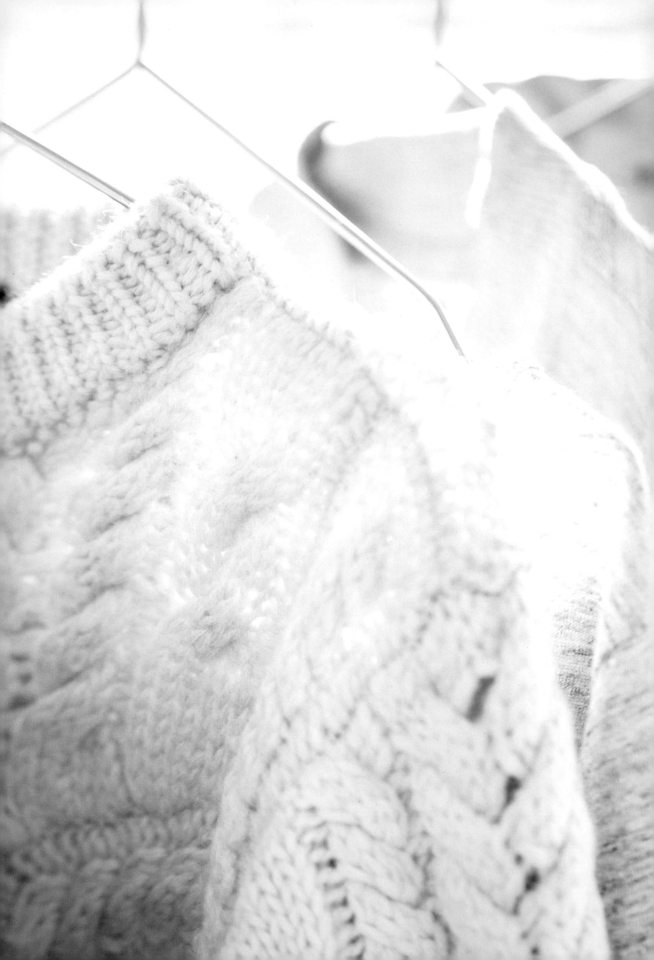

Things I like

OVERALL VIBE

Vintage

Seventies rock scene

Grown-up grunge

Maximalist

Folk style

INDIVIDUAL ITEMS

Leather jackets in all shapes and colors

Lace-up boots

Long knit cardigans over everything

Oversize seventies faux fur coat

Denim shirts

Colorful tunics with embroidery

COLORS

Black, black, and more black

Emerald green

All shades of purple

Gold (for jewelery and sequins)

Warm, rusty colors: bronze, auburn, amber, brick red

SILHOUETTES

High-rise skirts and pants

Palazzo pants

Jeans with ripped knees

Bodycon maxi dresses

Flowy caftans and tunics

Flared jeans

Crop tops with high-waisted skirts or pants

Long-line cardigans over minidresses, worn with knee-high boots

MATERIALS

Lace detailing

Eyelet pattern

Broken-in denim

Embroidery

All-over sequins

Corduroy

Velvet

Chunky knit sweaters, dresses, and cardigans

STYLING

Stacked bracelets

Long, layered necklaces

Thick belts

Lots and lots of layers

Cross-body bags

Cat-eye makeup

Long, flowy hair

Wide-brim hats

Double denim

Fringed bags

Flannel tied around hips

05 / Discover your style, phase II: Experiment and fine-tune

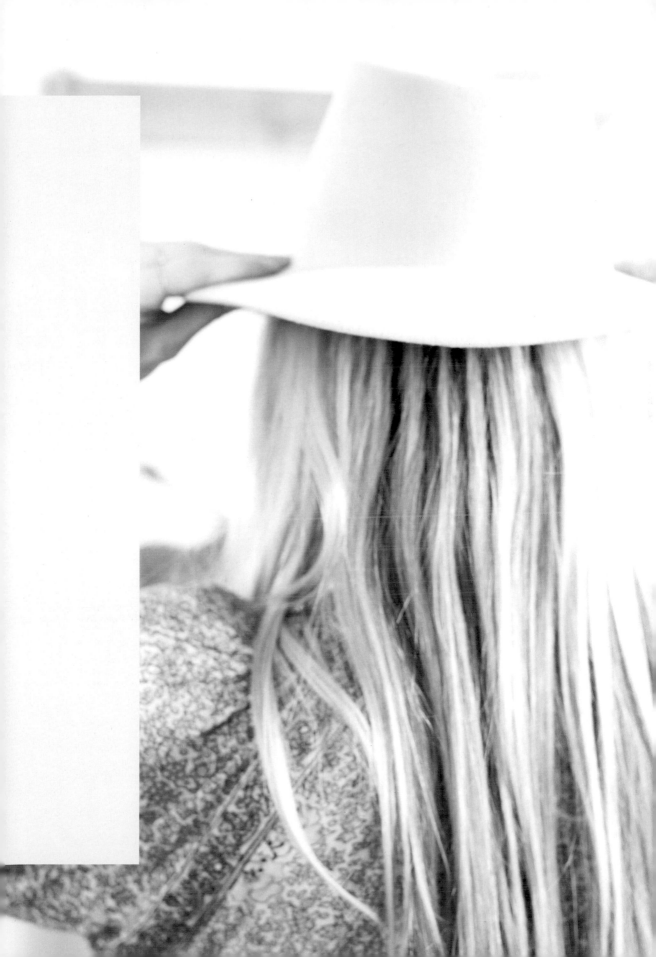

After all that research, it's time to get out into the field! Hit the stores, try stuff on, and experiment, experiment, experiment.

If you have just completed the inspiration phase and spent an afternoon sifting through magazines, blogs, and Pinterest, your head is now probably bursting with outfit ideas, colors, combinations, and fabrics to try. And hopefully you now also have at least a rough mental image of what your own personal style could look like. And that is great, but don't go rushing out to the shops just yet! That mental image is still just a preliminary draft because so far it's based purely on what kind of clothes you love and don't love—on other people.

But there is a big difference between appreciating a certain aesthetic on other people and loving that aesthetic on yourself.

Personally, I love the idea of empire-waist dresses with lace detailing, but I've never really liked how they look on me, so I just admire them from afar and stick to my go-to high-waisted skirts and camisoles in the summer.

There is a good chance that among all of the things you were drawn to as you collected inspiration, there are a few items on your list that belong in the "appreciate" category rather than the "wear" category. But unless you try it, you'll never know.

And that's why you need to experiment: to figure out not only exactly what type of aesthetic and specific pieces you like to wear, but also *how* you like to wear them. What type of top goes best with that type of skirt, how can you make that silhouette work on your body, what neckline do you prefer for sweaters, what styling tricks make you feel the most confident, and so on?

So take that list of pieces, colors, and outfit ideas that you wrote at the end of your inspiration search, and put it to the test. Make it your mission to try on every single thing on that list. For example, if you found yourself really drawn

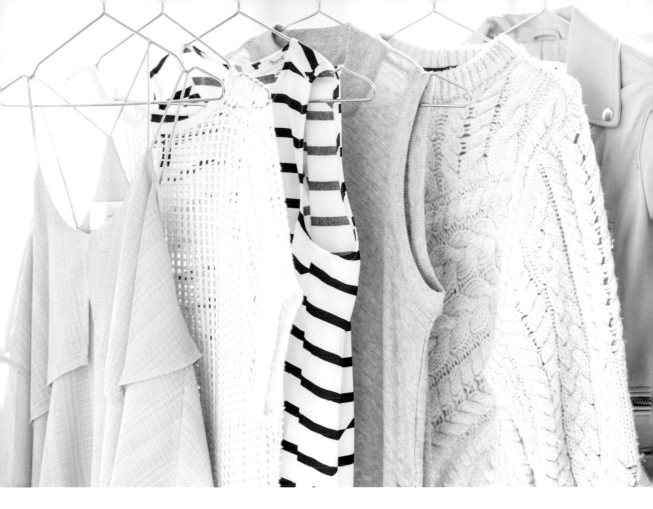

to A-line midi skirts, find a store that carries them (ideally in different versions) and just try them on, no strings attached. If one of the items on your list is "berry shades," try on every plum and raspberry piece you can find. Or, if you fell in love with an overall aesthetic, like a mod sixties look, challenge yourself to re-create that aesthetic using actual pieces you can find in a store.

Pretend you are a researcher conducting an experiment: keep an open mind, be sure to pay attention to every detail, snap pictures on your phone, and take lots and lots of notes.

Your goal here is to refine and improve the list you created during your inspiration session and end up with a comprehensive inventory of all the things you love plus lots of helpful details about how you like to wear individual pieces, your favorite combinations, fits to avoid, and so on. Try on as many pieces as you can get your hands on, but don't buy anything just yet.

Things I like—revised

Here's an example of what your list of elements may look like after you've done some experimenting:

OVERALL VIBE

Carrie Bradshaw inspired

Sophisticated glam

+ Immaculate tailoring

INDIVIDUAL ITEMS

A-line skirts

sling-back heels !!!

Pleated skirts

Fitted blazers

~~Mary Jane heels~~

~~Gingham pants~~ *better: gingham shirts*

COLORS

Champagne

Aquamarine blue *and other bright blues*

Soft pink *must be cool-toned!*

Dark-wash denim

Polka-dot pattern

~~All-white outfit~~

Floral patterns *should look glam instead of romantic/ whimsical, a large-scale pattern works best*

SILHOUETTES

Fitted pencil skirts with looser-fitting blouses *always tuck in blouse*

A-line skirts

Spaghetti-strap tops *new favorite combo*

Cowl-neck sweater

Slim-fitting jeans

For sweaters and shirts: V-neck

MATERIALS

Tulle (for skirts)

~~Ruffles~~ *no*

Silk shirts

Cashmere (for sweaters)

also great: merino wool

STYLING

Cuffed blazer sleeves

Chiffon scarfs

Thin belt around waistline *ALWAYS*

Delicate silver jewelry

~~Clutch bags~~

Thin belt over open cardigan

True red nail polish

~~Pearl necklaces~~ *too preppy for my taste, wear pearl earrings instead*

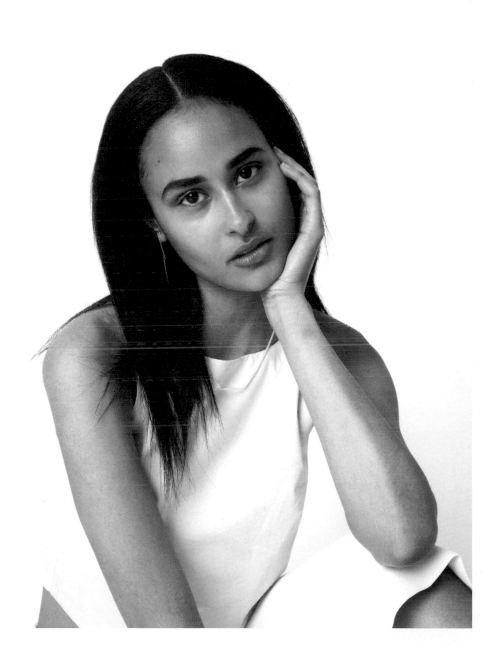

A word about finding clothes to try on

The best place to conduct your style experiment is a big department store, city center, or any place with lots of different stores and brands for you to sample. If you feel iffy about trying on stuff without actually buying something, remember that you do have the intention of buying something eventually, just not today. It's your right as customer to fully compare all your options before you make an informed purchasing decision. And once you have found your style and a brand that aligns well with your specific likes and dislikes, the store will be glad to have you.

Alternatively, you can ask friends and family to let you browse their wardrobes and sample a few of their pieces. And if several of your friends are also currently working on their personal style, you could even host a swap party, where everyone brings a selection of their own clothes for the others to try on.

How to assess your pieces

Whether it's a concrete piece like a pair of lace-up ballerina flats, a color combination like peach and sand, or an overall aesthetic you want to try out, throughout the experimentation phase, you'll inevitably come across some things you love right off the bat, some that you like but don't love, and others that just aren't working. Here's what to do in any of those scenarios.

YOU LOVE IT

Awesome! Write down every detail you can think of that makes this look work and don't forget to take a picture of your whole outfit so you have something to refer to later on.

YOU HATE IT

If you instantly hate something you've been really excited to try, it may feel like a total deal breaker, but, really, this is where the fun begins! Remember, building great outfits is a skill. And by trying something new, whether it's a color, silhouette, or overall look, you are venturing out into unknown territory. In other words, you can't expect to nail it on the first try.

Let's say you've been wanting to re-create a look you repeatedly found yourself drawn to while collecting inspiration: a high-waisted maxi skirt worn with a cropped top. So you find two pieces in a shop and go straight to the dressing rooms to try on your ensemble, expecting to have found a new go-to look . . . but then, once you catch the first glimpse of yourself in the mirror, you just feel disappointed. The whole outfit looks wrong, shapeless, and not at all like the modern seventies look that you were going for.

Should you scrap your maxi-skirt-plus-cropped-top idea for good and accept that that look just doesn't suit you? Not yet! Try the following instead.

Isolate the problem

This is key! Figure out exactly what element of the color, combination, silhouette, and so on isn't working. Be super specific about this. Because chances are, the problem isn't the overall idea you are testing (in this case the maxi skirt + cropped top combo) but the execution. Perhaps the cropped top is too long or not fitted enough to create the specific silhouette you are after. Perhaps the construction of the skirt doesn't fit the individual contours of your body. Perhaps the fabric is too thin and clingy. And maybe you just don't like the color of the top or the zipper detailing on the skirt, and it's distracting you. These are all things you can easily fix just by finding different pieces to create your look.

But what if the problem really does lie in the specific idea you are testing? Then you have two options.

Option 1: Tone down the intensity

If something really isn't working, the easiest way to still incorporate some of its overall vibe into your look is to simply wear it in smaller doses or in a toned-down format. For example, if going full on rock chic isn't your thing after all, you could try pairing your regular basics with a studded clutch bag and/or a leather jacket.

See page 71 for some more examples of how to tone down the intensity of something, depending on what type of element we are talking about.

Option 2: Scrap the idea

As you work through your list of ideas, you'll inevitably come across some elements or looks that you just cannot make work. Not everything that you love conceptually will translate well into outfits that fit your life. And some things you may just love on other people but not on yourself. And that's okay; no hard feelings. Simply make a note of it and move on.

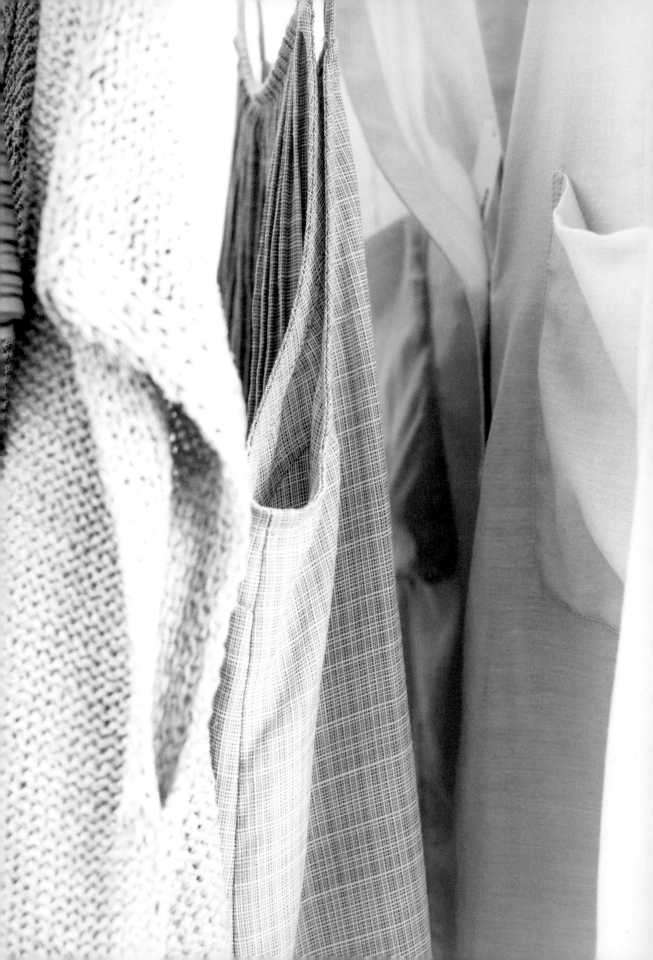

Making a look work for you

	IF THIS IS TOO MUCH...	TRY THIS	
		LOWER INTENSITY	SMALLER DOSE
OVERALL VIBE	printed maxi dresses, tie-dye, and bell-bottoms	flared jeans and tunics	single, superbohemian piece (like a headband) paired with more neutral basics
INDIVIDUAL ITEMS	knee-high lace-up boots	lace-up ankle boots	
COLORS	fuscia pink top	top in a softer rose shade	smaller doses of fuscia (nail color or a single piece of jewelry)
SILHOUETTES	oversized shirt with wide-leg pants	that same shirt with straight-cut pants and a belt to break up the silhouette	
MATERIALS	velvet blazer	velvet purse	
	lace dress	cotton dress with a lace hemline	
STYLING	bold wing of eyeliner	subtle flick of eyeliner	
	multilayered pearl necklace	pearl earrings	

YOU LIKE IT . . . BUT DON'T LOVE IT

Almost! Perhaps something about your outfit looks a little off, or you are just not crazy about it. In either case, you can follow the same process here as for looks and elements you hate: isolate the problem and fix it, see if you like it in a toned-down format, or scrap it. Chances are, if you like 80 percent of a look, a little tweaking can easily turn that into 100 percent.

How to translate an overall aesthetic into an outfit

Test-driving an overall aesthetic, whether it's something that's relatively defined (like a grungy nineties look) or your own concoction (like "beachy retro chic"), can be a little trickier than simply trying on a specific piece or color, because it involves an extra step: figuring out how to translate that overall vibe into a wearable outfit.

The easiest way to do this is to choose two or three inspiration images that best convey the overall vibe you are trying to re-create, put them side by side, and try to pick out just a few concrete elements that stand out, like a color, a specific piece, or a silhouette. What do all the images have in common? What one thing really signifies that overall feeling that all the images share? Then, build an outfit around those elements.

Extra challenges

Wanna score some brownie points? Complete these extra challenges as part of your style experiment:

- List three things you love on other people but think you could never pull off yourself. Go on a mission to make them work on you by trying out lots of different versions or toning down the intensity.
- Go into a store that you consider to be totally not your style and challenge yourself to find one complete outfit that you would actually wear.

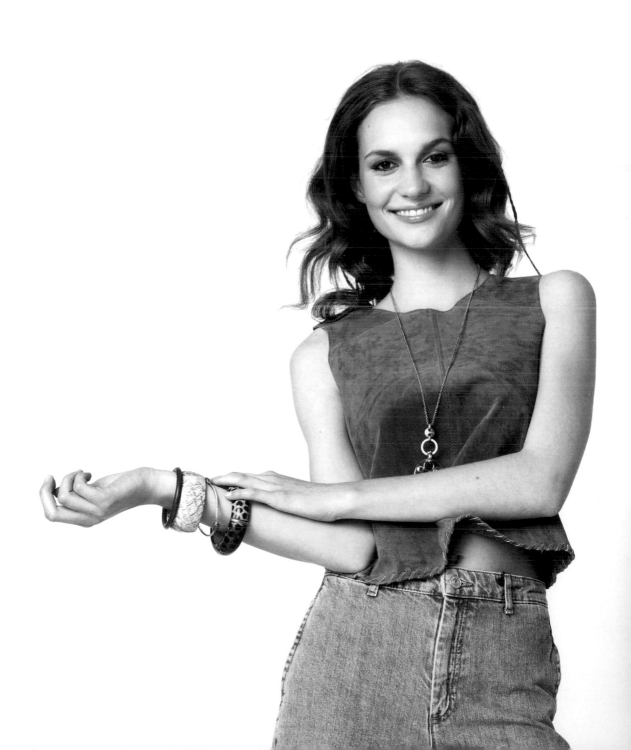

ARE YOU UNCOMFORTABLE OR JUST OUT OF YOUR COMFORT ZONE?

As you experiment and venture out into new style territory, you may at times feel a little nervous and unsure about new pieces, cuts, and colors, especially if the new style you are test-driving is bolder or more out-there than what you are used to. If you are trying to revamp your style, feeling out of your comfort zone is actually a good sign, because your comfort zone may have been safe but it didn't make you happy. If something truly is your style, it's just a matter of time until you warm up to it and feel great. In short, being a little out of your comfort zone is natural and nothing to worry about. But at the beginning, it may feel dangerously similar to feeling just plain uncomfortable with something because you truly don't like it, and you may end up dismissing a great piece that could have been a new wardrobe favorite.

To prevent that, you need to learn how to tell the difference between being out of your comfort zone and feeling uncomfortable because a particular piece or outfit just isn't working.

Feeling out of your comfort zone has nothing to do with your personal style and everything to do with your confidence levels.

Essentially, when you are out of your comfort zone, there are two forces pulling you in opposite directions. Your (much more objective) eye for style is telling you, "Yep, I love it, let's wear it," but your confidence center is telling you, "Hm, I don't know, isn't it a little too risqué for work? I've never worn all white before. . . . Isn't my butt a little too much on display? Will people stare?"

Fortunately, confidence levels vary on a day-to-day basis, and so one way to reduce the chance of low confidence distorting your perception of a new piece is to simply complete your style experiment on days when you are already in a good mood. Don't go faux shopping if you're not feeling well, you're stressed, or you're exhausted. Instead, pick a day when you can relax, after you have gotten a good night's sleep and had time to do your hair and makeup. Make sure you feel good *before* you hit the shops. An overall positive attitude is going to make it much easier to not let those nagging (and completely unneccessary voices) get in the way of you and great style.

A second way to distinguish between being out of your comfort zone and simply not liking a piece is to trick your confidence center into shutting down temporarily with a little thought experiment. For example, let's say you have always been a jeans-and-T-shirt kinda gal but are now trying on a simple dress for the first time and feeling really strange. Ask yourself, if a fairy godmother gave me total confidence and zapped all my body hang-ups, would I wear this? Or, if I moved to a new city and had the chance to completely reinvent myself, would I wear this? If the answer is yes, you can feel optimistic that this type of piece aligns well with your unique aesthetic and you will eventually get used to it and wear it with pride.

If you love something, like a bright color or a specific pattern, but not as part of your wardrobe, see if you can incorporate it into your life in other ways! For example, I'm a big fan of wild floral patterns, but rather than wearing them, I reserve them for home decor and artwork.

Playing pretend helps you move past your natural but temporary insecurities to get down to what really matters: your true feelings about that dress. It sounds silly, but it really works. Try it!

And don't forget: you don't have to dive right into the deep end and dress head-to-toe in black leather and studs, even if that's what you ultimately want. You can start by dipping your toes in and slowly easing into your new style—by wearing a single edgier piece with your go-to basics, for example.

Create your own rules: Building a fit and fabric guide

You already know I am not a fan of fashion rules that tell you what to wear based on your body shape, coloring, or answers to a handful of multiple-choice questions. But I do believe rules can be helpful—as long as you set them for yourself. For example, one of my personal style rules is that I don't wear tops that aren't fitted around the waist or don't look good when tucked into pants. This is not because of my body shape, but just because I've learned from experience that I just always prefer some definition around my hips or waist. Now that I know that, I can safely skip things like empire-waist tops or long-line chunky knit sweaters while I am out shopping, which saves time and energy.

Having rules is especially helpful when it comes to fabrics and fits, because these are hard to get right, can make or break an outfit, and on top of that, strongly depend on your personal preferences. But again, to uncover your personal preferences, you first need to do a fair bit of experimenting. And the experimentation phase is the perfect opportunity to do just that!

Below and on the next page you'll find a list of the most common fabrics, materials, and fit elements, such as sleeve length, necklines, and so on. As you go along and try on lots of different clothes, take a moment to assess how much you like both the fabric and the fit of the piece you are currently trying on and make a note of it in your style file. If you already know for a fact that you hate or love some of the things on the list, feel free to enter that before shopping, but for everything you aren't 100 percent sure about, don't knock it till you've tried it.

FABRICS AND MATERIALS

- Angora
- Cashmere
- Chambray
- Chiffon
- Corduroy
- Cotton
- Denim
- Faux fur
- Faux leather
- Fleece
- Knits
- Leather
- Linen
- Mohair
- Polyester
- Raw denim
- Rayon
- Satin
- Silk
- Spandex
- Suede
- Tweed
- Velvet
- Viscose
- Wool

FITS

Necklines

- Boat neck
- Cowl neck
- Crew neck
- Deep V-neck
- Halter neck
- Scoop neck
- Square neck
- Sweetheart neckline
- Turtleneck
- V-neck

Sleeves

- Cap sleeves
- Dolman
- Half length
- Off the shoulder
- Raglan
- Short
- Sleeveless
- Spaghetti straps
- Strapless
- Three-quarter length

Waistlines (tops and dresses)

- A-line
- Drop waist
- Empire
- Fitted, but not tight
- Loose fitting
- Slim fitting
- Straight
- Tailored

Dress/skirt length

- Above knee
- Knee length
- Maxi
- Mid length
- Mini

Skirt type

- A-line
- Fitted
- Full
- Pleated
- Straight

Trouser length

- Ankle length
- Full length
- Hot pants
- Knee length
- Mid thigh
- Short
- Three-quarter length

Trouser type

- Boot cut
- Boyfriend
- Chinos
- Flared
- Harem
- Pleated
- Skintight/legging fit
- Slim fitting
- Tailored
- Tapered

06/

Putting it all together: Your style profile

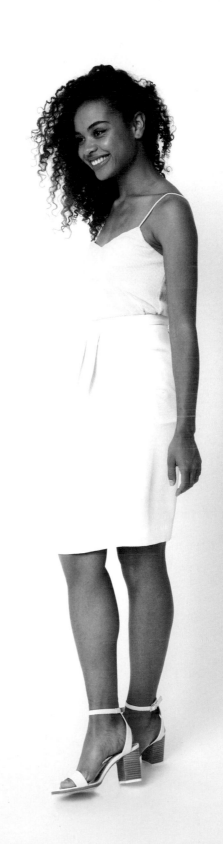

Congratulations! You've done the work and spent time in dressing rooms sampling new styles, fits, and materials. You are now ready to take all that information and weave everything into one coherent story line: your personal style.

After completing your fieldwork, you are now hopefully at a place where you have a pretty good idea of what kinds of cuts, colors, and combinations you love, how you like things to fit, and what overall style you feel most comfortable in.

This chapter is about synthesizing all those findings and turning everything into a detailed profile of your *ideal* style.

Regardless of what's currently in your wardrobe, having a clear picture of how you ideally would like to dress is a good idea because it gives you a concrete road map that you can use to tweak, upgrade, or overhaul your wardrobe step by step.

Style profile overview

In this chapter, you'll learn how to put together a style profile that consists of two parts:

- Part 1: A mood board that expresses the overall feeling of your style
- Part 2: A written summary of the key qualities of your style

Why two parts? Because your style profile needs to fulfill two crucial criteria: it has to be inspiring *and* practical. The mood board covers the visual, bigger-picture perspective of your style, while your written summary acts as a road map for implementing it.

One word before we get started: at this point, it's totally natural to feel a little intimidated and worry about whether you are even ready to pinpoint your personal style, much less write a detailed profile of it. But remember: when it comes to personal style, nothing is ever set in stone. In a few years you will probably shake your head at some of your current favorite pieces. Your style is ever evolving, but that doesn't mean there's no point in building a wardrobe that you love right now. Developing a great sense of style is all about practice. So don't worry if you aren't 100 percent sure you've discovered your personal style yet. Even if you don't end up implementing every little part of your style profile or change your mind about some things, aiming for a coherent overall aesthetic will already do wonders for your wardrobe and help you train your eye for style. Bottom line: Even if you don't feel completely ready yet, simply give it your best shot, and revise it as you go along.

Ready? Okay, let's go!

Find the pattern: A first sketch of your personal style

Before you start working on the two parts of your style profile, it's important that you understand the overall feeling of your style and its main components.

Now, hopefully, during your style research and fieldwork, you already noticed patterns among your favorite pieces, colors, materials, and silhouettes. Perhaps you were drawn primarily to structured, minimalist outfits, clean lines, and jewel tones. Or you noticed you love everything with a romantic vintage vibe from floral patterns to lace detailings. Or maybe you discovered you feel best when mixing two styles that don't have much in common at first sight, like a sporty, urban look with a touch of punk.

If so, this step will be easy for you. If you didn't notice any patterns, now is your chance to look over all of your different likes again and figure out how everything fits together.

Here's how: Go back over the final list of elements that you put together during your experimentation phase and answer the questions below. Write full sentences or just bullet points, whatever you like. Use your inspiration material and any pictures you took of yourself during your fieldwork as a visual reference. Go back and forth as much as you need to until you feel you have a good grasp of the main idea of your style. Focus on the big-picture idea only; don't worry about details yet. You'll get a chance to fine-tune those when you create your style profile.

- What is the overall feeling of this style?
- What are the most important individual pieces?
- What are the most important colors?
- What are the most important silhouettes, cuts, and fits?
- Are there any fabrics or materials that are essential to this style?
- Are there any styling tricks that are essential to this style?
- Write down several concrete ways that two or more of the above elements could be combined within a single outfit.

Here are some examples:

Denim (material) + lace (material) + minidress (silhouette) =
Wear denim jacket over a short dress with a lace hemline.

Modern bohemian (overall vibe) + jumpsuit (individual piece) + olive green (color) =
Wear an olive green jumpsuit with platform heels, a beaded clutch bag, and chandelier earrings.

MERGING TWO DIFFERENT STYLES

Is it possible to merge two styles that don't have anything in common? This is a really common question, and the answer is yes, it is definitely possible to combine two aesthetics into one coherent style. In fact, that's what defining your own personal style is about: pinpointing your exact likes and figuring out a way to weave them into a story line and a unique look that is completely your own.

Now, the reason this may seem like a tricky job at first is because we are all so used to classifying outfits and style elements as bohemian, preppy, classic, minimalist, French-chic, and so on. We think "a fitted waistline plus a flared, midlength skirt" equals a fifties look and that "clean lines plus a monochrome color palette plus no accessories" equals minimal. Styles like these are to the fashion world what baroque, art deco, or impressionism are to the art world: very distinct visual concepts that are usually tied to a certain cultural movement or era and can be clearly identified by a set of characteristics. But for the purpose of developing your own style, you absolutely do not have to stay within those predefined lines.

If you think about it, a style is nothing but a set of individual elements. To merge two different aesthetics, you need to break them up into their elements, carefully select exactly which of these you want to incorporate into your own style concept, and then figure out how to turn them into actual outfits.

Let's say you love a minimalist look but are also inspired by the nineties grunge scene. As a first step, you need to ask yourself which exact elements—colors, shapes, textures, specific pieces, details, and so on—of those two styles you want to be a part of your own unique look. By doing this, you are reducing those big, restrictive top-level concepts into a simple set of tangible elements that are much easier to work with. Nineties grunge and minimalism may not sound very compatible, but a sleek pair of tailored pants worn with a heavy leather jacket definitely does.

Style profile part 1: The mood board

Building mood boards is a simple and yet oh-so-powerful creative technique that's used by everyone from fashion editors to graphic designers to architects.

Essentially, a mood board is nothing but a collection of images on a canvas. But because of the total freedom you have in arranging your images and the ability to see all your inspiration in one place, mood boards are a great way to visualize abstract, creative ideas and narratives, whether that is the overall feeling of a branding campaign, a fashion collection, or your personal style.

Building a mood board is just as much about the process as the outcome. Your goal is to end up with something that you can use as a complete visual reference to your style, but the act of choosing images and arranging them will also help you get a feeling for how all the different elements work with each other and ensure that you really love the overall picture you have created.

To create your mood board, you'll be using all your favorite images from your inspiration search, so make sure you have those on hand for these next steps.

CHOOSING A FORMAT FOR YOUR MOOD BOARD

There are three ways to build a mood board.

Analog

Do it old-school: print out images or cut them out of magazines and then glue everything onto a big piece of cardboard. If you are the crafty type and enjoy this type of stuff, this is a great option because it allows you to truly engage with your images. Just make sure you have access to a printer so you aren't limited to choosing only what you can find in print.

Digital 1

My go-to method for creating a mood board is to collect all the images digitally and then use an app or software to arrange them all. Depending on your tech skills, you can go super fancy with this and build your mood board on Photoshop or InDesign, but any other program that allows you to create free-form collages works just as well, so just pick the one with which you are most comfortable.

The major advantage of this method over the analog one is that it's faster because you don't have to print out your inspiration images first and can easily resize images to give them more or less visual impact on the overall mood board.

Digital 2

If you don't want to bother with graphic programs or are strapped for time you can also simply collect all your images in a folder on your computer or on Pinterest. Beware: This is the quickest but also the least effective option because it doesn't allow you to arrange your images or alter their size, so therefore you'll be somewhat limited in regard to accurately portraying your style.

SELECTING PICTURES FOR YOUR MOOD BOARD

Once you have chosen a format for your mood board, you can start selecting images for it. The key thing to keep in mind here is that you want to use images that (1) cover all the *individual* components you want to be the foundation of your style, like colors, materials, and so on and (2) accurately represent the *overall* feeling of the look you are going for when viewed as a whole. The easiest way to meet both criteria is to focus on them one by one, starting with the individual components of your style: take your list of colors, themes, silhouettes, styling techniques, and materials and then find a picture that best represents each one of them. For many of these, you will be able to use the original images you collected during your inspiration search, but if you discovered any important caveats (for example, "wear white only for accessories"), make sure you find a new picture to represent that. Also, if you took any pictures of yourself wearing outfits or individual pieces during your fieldwork, feel free to include these as well.

FINE-TUNING YOUR MOOD BOARD

Now that you have chosen all the individual components of your mood board, it's time to arrange them on your canvas in a way that best reflects the overall style you have in mind. To do that, you need to (1) decide how important each of the individual aspects of your style are and (2) give them a proportionate amount of space on your mood board. Some colors, silhouettes, or materials will be absolutely essential to the overall feeling of your style, while others are nice add-ons but not quite as crucial.

Emphasize ideas and elements that really signify your style by giving them a center spot, using bigger photos, and/or including several different examples of the same idea. Put specific pieces and side ideas toward the edges.

Keep fine-tuning your mood board until it represents the exact aesthetic you are going for. Add images, take some away, tweak, tweak, and tweak. Then continue with the second part of your style profile.

Style profile part 2: The written summary

 The purpose of writing a summary of your style once you have finished your mood board is to give you something concrete and tangible to refer to as you tailor your wardrobe to your style.

To create your written summary, use your notes from the inspiration and fieldwork stage, as well as your mood board, to answer the questions on page 87.

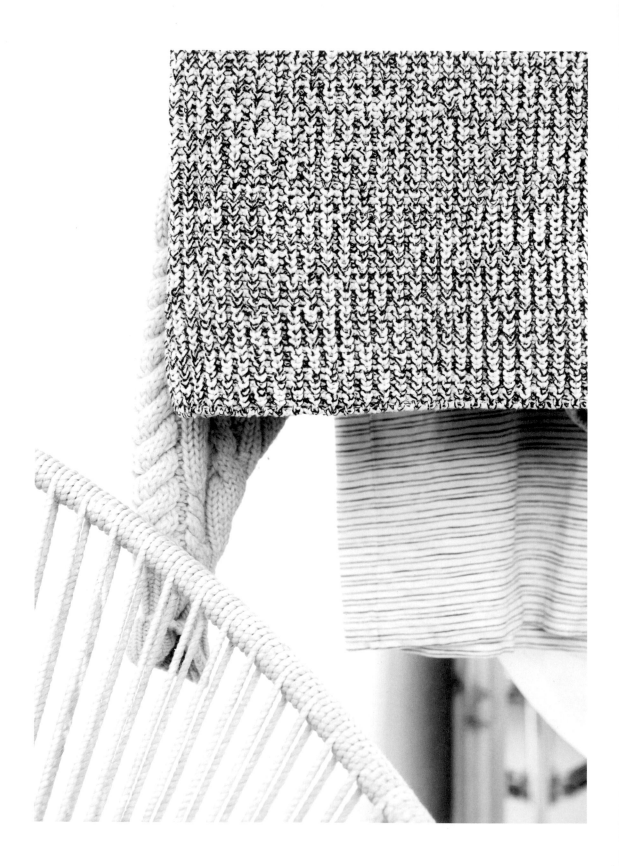

STYLE QUESTIONS

- What's the best name for your personal style?
- In one or two sentences, what's the overall idea behind your style?
- What does a typical outfit look like for this style?
- What does this style say about its wearer? What three character qualities does it convey?
- What are the key pieces of this style?
- What are the dominant colors?
- Which silhouettes, cuts, and fits are a part of this style?
- What type of materials and fabrics work well with this style?
- What does the styling look like? Think accessories, specific styling techniques, and hair and makeup.

Naming Your Style

Not sure what to call your personal style? Here's some inspiration:

- West Coast casual meets East Coast prep
- Contemporary mod
- Classic menswear
- Grace Kelly goes to college
- Urban minimalism
- Eclectic high fashion on a budget
- Bohemian modern
- Hitchcock glam with a twist
- New York luxe
- Laid-back street style
- Colorful and cosmopolitan
- Twenty-first-century Victorian romantic

Remember: the name you choose for your style doesn't have to make sense to anyone but you. So feel free to get creative!

To give you a complete example of what such a written summary could look like, here's the style profile for the style Viktoria is modeling in this book:

Viktoria's Style

What's the best name for your personal style?

Menswear-inspired French chic.

In one or two sentences, what's the overall idea behind your style?

My personal style is based on understated, tailored separates, menswear-inspired staples, and a cool, light color palette. It looks effortless but ultra polished.

What does a typical outfit look like for this style?

A striped button-down shirt with tailored chinos or boyfriend jeans, oxfords, and a blazer.

What does this style say about its wearer? What three character qualities does it convey?

Confidence, sophistication, polish.

What are the key pieces of this style?

Black oxfords, loafers, button-down shirts, light-wash boyfriend jeans, and a navy blazer.

What are the dominant colors?

Shades of blue, sand, and white; no patterns or prints except stripes.

Which silhouettes, cuts, and fits are a part of this style?

Relaxed fits for tops and bottoms; chinos, jeans (skinny or boyfriend), and loose-fitting suit-style trousers. All pants must be high-waisted to add structure and definition. Tops are either crew neck or collared. Blazers and coats must be long-line, not too fitted.

What type of materials and fabrics work well with this style?

Thick cotton material for pants, jackets, and tops; linen for shirts and jackets; rough leather for belts and footwear; thick denim material with little stretch; chunky knits in winter, corduroy for fall, seersucker for spring and summer.

What does the styling look like? Think accessories, specific styling techniques, and hair and makeup.

Accessorize with slim leather belts, classic watches, or hats. Shirts are tucked into pants. Roll up hemlines of pants to show a peek of ankle. Makeup: Emphasize brows.

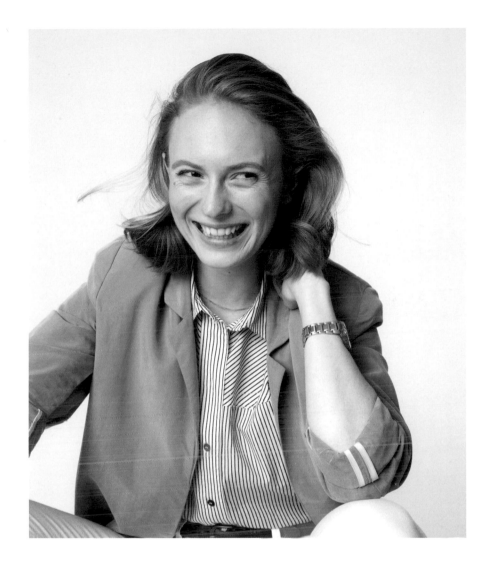

One Last Step

Once you are happy with your style profile, give yourself a pat on the back!
You've just completed the entire style-defining section of this book and are well
on your way to great personal style and the perfect wardrobe. Before you delve
straight into the practical part of the book and learn how to now translate your
newfound style into an expressive, versatile wardrobe, take a moment to
complete this one last step.

 Figure out in what ways your current wardrobe differs from your ideal
style. That will help you set priorities once you are ready to overhaul
your closet and choose a few new pieces.

PART III

BUILD YOUR DREAM WARDROBE

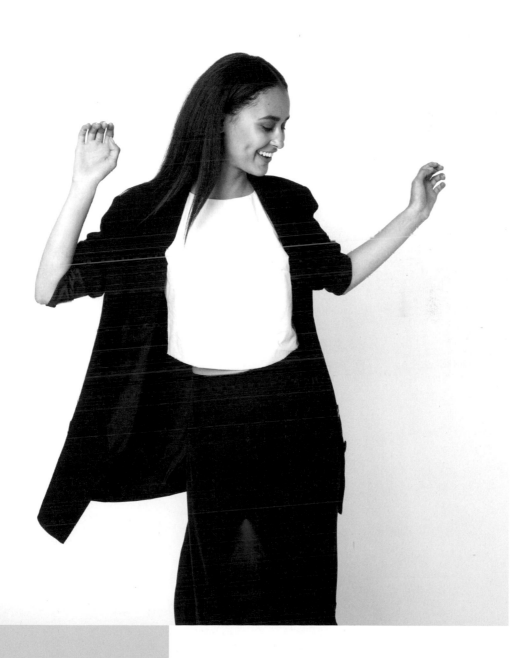

07/
Closet detox: The complete guide

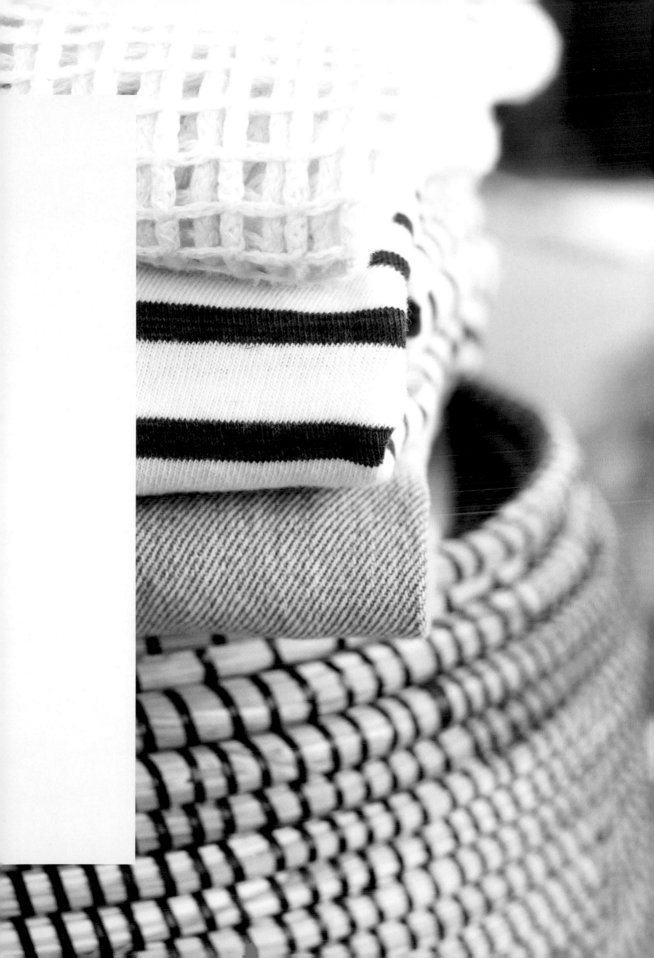

Clear the clutter and get your wardrobe in tip-top shape! Say good-bye to anything that doesn't reflect your personal style, still has its tag on, or does nothing for your confidence.

Okay, let's get down to business! Now that you have defined your personal style, you're ready to tackle your closet head on and transform it into your best wardrobe yet. In this section, we'll use your style profile as a road map to revamp your current wardrobe and figure out exactly what type of pieces should go on your shopping list. But first, we have to do a little prep work, starting with a big closet detox in this chapter.

Think of your closet like a house that needs a top-to-bottom renovation. Before you can paint the walls and install new floors, you need to strip off that ugly wallpaper, tear up the old carpet, and get rid of broken, rusty hardware. In the end you may well discover that all your wardrobe needs is a fresh coat of paint and some new light fixtures. But first, you need to get rid of all the clutter to see exactly what you're working with.

Once your wardrobe is in good shape, maintain it with a biannual mini detox. Read more about wardrobe maintenance in chapter 21.

Your goal for this chapter is to go through your entire wardrobe and get rid of everything that doesn't reflect your style or that you haven't worn in a long time. Be thorough here: now is the time to sort through all those piles of clothes that have been sitting at the back of your closet for months and part with impulse buys and anything that feels itchy, doesn't fit right, or doesn't fit into your style profile. Reserve at least a full afternoon or evening for uninterrupted detox time.

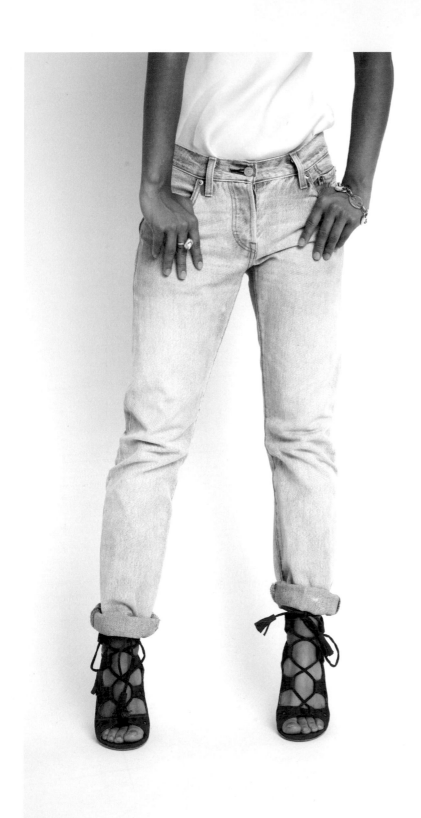

Pre-detox prep

WHAT YOU NEED:

- One or two trash bags
- Six boxes (or bags)
- A full-length mirror
- A camera (your phone's is fine)
- Some good music, snacks, and stamina

LABEL YOUR SIX BOXES LIKE THIS:

- Donate or sell
- Keepsakes
- Trial separation
- Get tailored
- Repair
- Off-season storage

All done? Ok, then turn on your music and let's get cracking!

The detox

Pick up each piece in your wardrobe one by one and use the flow chart on pages 100–101 to thoroughly assess how you feel about it and determine its fate.

PIECES THAT AREN'T WORKING OUT

Donate or sell

Any item that doesn't reflect your personal style, is way too uncomfortable, or does nothing for your confidence doesn't deserve a spot in your wardrobe. But if the piece is still in good condition, there's no reason to let it become landfill! Donate your pieces to a charity shop, give them to a friend who may like them, or sell them to make a little extra cash.

Keepsakes

Your graduation dress, the shoes you wore at your wedding, or the beaded bag you bought on a once-in-a-lifetime trip to India—pieces that you have stopped wearing long ago but that remind you of a special, happy time, can be impossible to part with. And the good news is, you don't have to. Just make sure you treat those pieces for what they are—keepsakes that deserve a place somewhere in your home, but not in your closet. Collect pieces that have a sentimental value for you in the keepsakes box for now and then find a good permanent spot for them once you've completed the detox.

Trash bag

Anything that's stained, ripped, or otherwise broken beyond repair belongs in the trash, no exceptions. The same goes for worn-out underwear, socks, and exercise gear.

PIECES YOU AREN'T SURE ABOUT

Trial separation

A great way to reveal your true feelings about pieces you are not sure about is to store them outside of your closet in a separate box for a while, perhaps under your bed. That way, if you truly miss an item, you can easily retrieve it, but chances are, you'll forget about most of the stuff in there after a couple of weeks and can then confidently get rid of them.

Back in your closet (for now)

If your wardrobe needs a major revamp, you may well feel tempted to just throw out the majority of your clothes during your detox because they just don't work with your newfound style. Don't! If you get rid of too much now, you'll likely be left with a big gap in your closet that you will want to fill ASAP. And that gap may tempt you to buy way too much stuff too soon, before you have gotten the chance to think it through. And then you'll be back at square one. Do this instead: just for now, keep items that you feel only so-so about, as long as you still wear them regularly (at least once every two weeks). Don't throw out your go-to pair of work pants, even if they don't really reflect your ideal style or could fit a little better. The same goes for your trusty but worn-out sweater and your one nude strapless bra that's taken on a gray tinge over the years but is your only option for white tops. You can always replace these later on. But at this stage, while your wardrobe still needs a lot of work, thoughtfully spending your money on missing key pieces and other essentials will have a much bigger impact.

Get tailored

Shortening hemlines, taking in a baggy shirt, or adding darts—there are a lot of things a good tailor can do to improve the fit and silhouette of a piece and that don't cost a fortune. Put pieces you would wear if the fit were improved in the tailor box, and take them to a tailor after you're done with the detox.

PIECES YOU LOVE

Repair

Always keep a mini sewing kit on hand so you can take care of basic repairs yourself, like fixing undone seams or loose buttons. For trickier jobs, like taking in a waist, it's usually better to get a professional on the case.

Off-season storage

This one is optional, but consider creating some extra breathing room in your closet by storing off-season clothes somewhere else. I personally prefer to reserve every inch of my closet space for pieces that are an active part of my wardrobe right now, this season. I store all my off-season pieces, like chunky knit sweaters in the summer or strappy tops and dresses in the winter, outside of my actual closet, in a couple of boxes underneath my bed. That way, when I open my closet in the morning, I see only things I could actually wear today, and my closet is much less cluttered.

Back in your closet

Hooray! If a piece fits your personal style, makes you feel confident and comfortable, and you can already think of several different ways to wear it, it's a keeper!

Post-detox to-dos

 Once you have gone through your entire wardrobe piece by piece, you'll have a super clear overview of your closet. Use that clarity to do a quick status analysis:

- What are obvious gaps in your closet?
- What type of pieces do you already have enough of?

Think item categories (T-shirts, jeans, semicasual work tops), colors, seasonal clothes, and function.

Write a quick paragraph summarizing your findings and first conclusions, like this:

The closet detox has once again confirmed that I like to shop for shoes more than anything else. Even now that I have gotten rid of every pair that I never wear or that doesn't work for my style, I still own more footwear than dresses, pants, and outerwear combined. Conclusion: I definitely don't need any more shoes for a while. What I do need are basic tops, jeans, and skirts, because the majority of my clothes are too statement-y to wear with anything other than plain pieces. I also need more clothes for work. Right now I have only two (!) pairs of pants that I can wear to the office that I actually like, and I spend forty hours a week there!

If I Paid for It, I'm Wearing It: The Sunk-Cost Fallacy

Do you hate wasting things? Are you the type of person who will go out to buy bread just so you can use up that left-over piece of cheese in the fridge, or force yourself to use up a bottle of shower gel, even though you hate the smell? If so you're prone to committing what is called the sunk-cost fallacy.

Sunk costs are sums that we have already paid and can't get back, that is, money spent on anything that isn't returnable. Because we are very loss averse and far more motivated by the possibility of losing things than the possibility of gaining things, sunk costs are pretty much the worst for us.

That's why we try to avoid them whenever we can, by forcing ourselves to "use up" whatever it is we paid for. We sit through a full two-hour movie we hate, even though there's a million other things we'd rather do. We continue eating long after the food stopped tasting good. And we refuse to get rid of clothes we dislike and stopped wearing, because we paid good money for them once upon a time and we don't want that investment to go to waste.

But that's exactly where the fallacy lies: The money is already spent, so there is nothing left to waste, except for your time, energy, and closet space. And remember: just because you don't like a piece, doesn't mean someone else won't love it! So find a new owner for it and move on.

Closet Detox

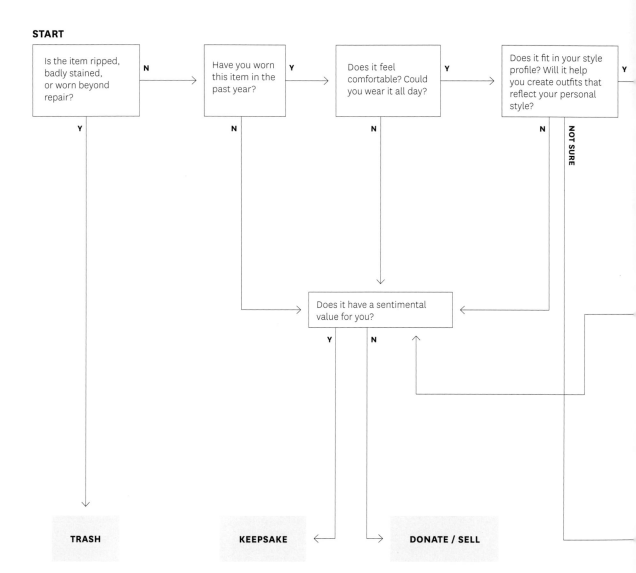

START

Is the item ripped, badly stained, or worn beyond repair?

N →

Have you worn this item in the past year?

Y →

Does it feel comfortable? Could you wear it all day?

Y →

Does it fit in your style profile? Will it help you create outfits that reflect your personal style?

Y →

Y ↓ (from first box)

N ↓ (from second box)

N ↓ (from third box)

N ↓ / NOT SURE (from fourth box)

Does it have a sentimental value for you?

Y ↓   N ↓

TRASH

KEEPSAKE

DONATE / SELL

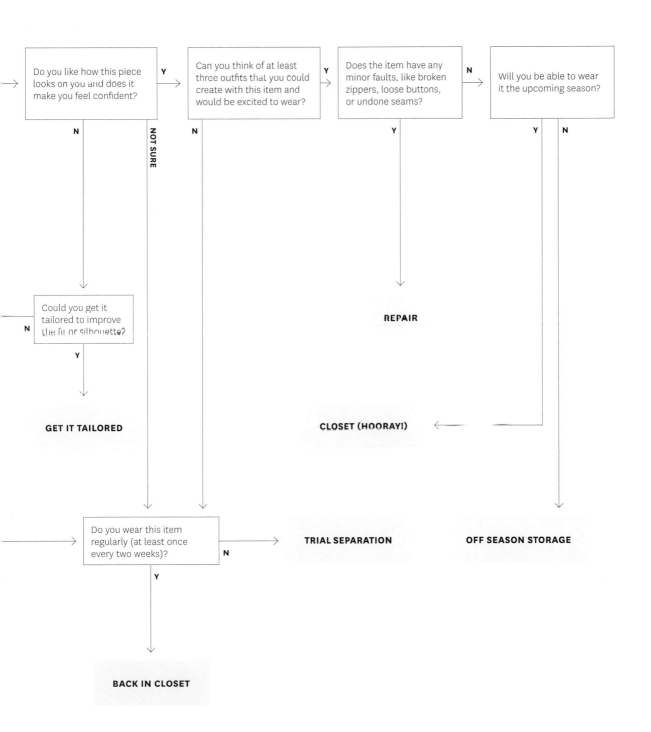

Do you like how this piece looks on you and does it make you feel confident? **Y** →

Can you think of at least three outfits that you could create with this item and would be excited to wear? **Y** →

Does the item have any minor faults, like broken zippers, loose buttons, or undone seams? **N** →

Will you be able to wear it the upcoming season?

N ↓   **NOT SURE**   **N** ↓   **Y** ↓   **Y**   **N**

Could you get it tailored to improve the fit or silhouette?

N   **Y** ↓

REPAIR

GET IT TAILORED

CLOSET (HOORAY!) ←

Do you wear this item regularly (at least once every two weeks)? **N** →

TRIAL SEPARATION

OFF SEASON STORAGE

Y ↓

BACK IN CLOSET

08/

How to build a wardrobe that fits your life

(not your fantasy life)

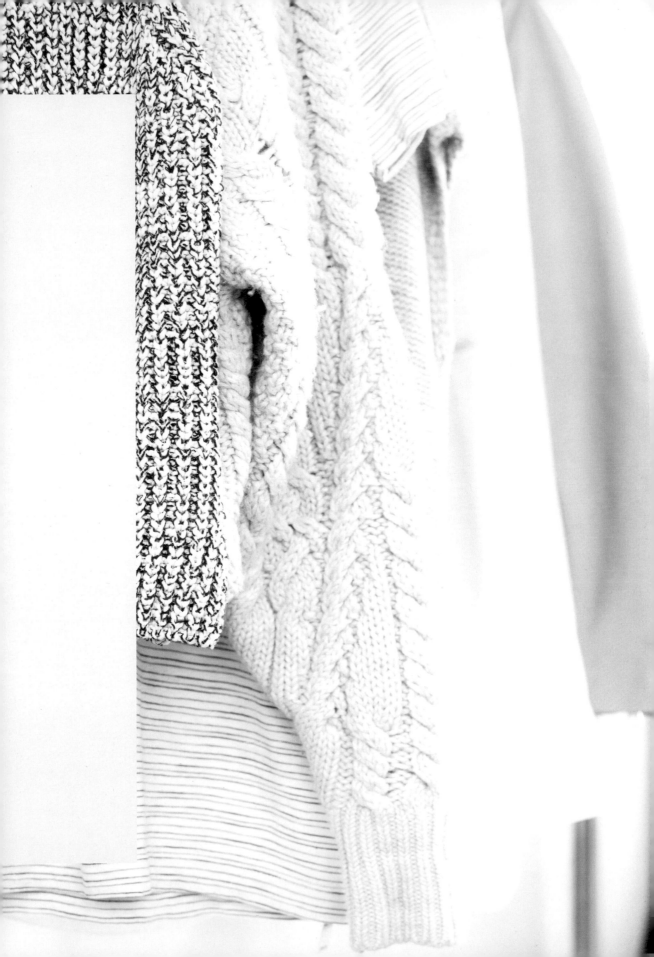

Repeat after me: Your dream closet should be tailored to your personal style *and* your lifestyle. You already know all about your personal style, now let's have a closer look at your lifestyle!

Fashion is a form of art, and you want your clothes to look good, sure, but you also need them to be *feel* good and be practical because you spend your life in them. You have stuff to do, places to go, and people to meet. A functional wardrobe is one that supports you in all these endeavours, rather than making your life harder.

If you work in an office only two days a week, a closet full of exquisitely tailored suits and little else is not what you need. And if you're a busy student who spends the majority of her time in the library, a bunch of pretty bikinis and going-out dresses aren't going to keep you well-dressed either.

To be functional, your wardrobe needs to be optimally tailored to your lifestyle, or in other words, what you are doing all day. Not what you would like to do, or what you will be doing sometime in the future, hopefully, if all goes well. But right now.

Of course, it's easy to see why so many of us end up with wardrobes that seem to be tailored to a life very different from our own: Some things are just more fun to buy than others!

It's more fun to browse the swimwear section of your favorite online shop and daydream about lounging at the beach than it is to think about what you'll wear during all those hours that you have to spend at the library with your nose buried in textbooks.

And yet, those study sessions are still going to happen and you can't go naked! So you might as well dress in a way that makes you feel confident and ready to tackle the day.

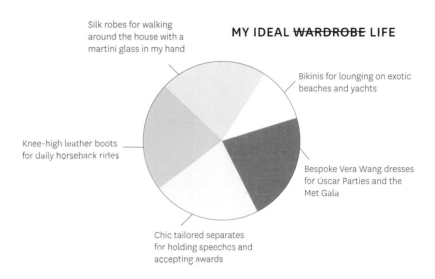

MY IDEAL ~~WARDROBE~~ LIFE

Silk robes for walking around the house with a martini glass in my hand

Bikinis for lounging on exotic beaches and yachts

Knee-high leather boots for daily horseback rides

Bespoke Vera Wang dresses for Oscar Parties and the Met Gala

Chic tailored separates for holding speeches and accepting awards

The perfect wardrobe for you is one that helps you do just that, no matter what your plans are. Ideally, it should match your lifestyle in terms of all the different activities you do on a regular basis, in roughly equal distributions. That means if you work in a corporate office full-time and go out to a fancy dinner twice a month, you should own considerably more work clothes than fancy evening clothes. If you work out three times a week and make it to the beach once a year, you should have more gym clothes than bathing suits. Makes sense, right?

You don't have to get super specific with this and work out the exact number of outfits you need for activity X and so on (although you totally can, if that's your thing). But, as you prepare to overhaul your wardrobe, it's helpful to at least have a good idea of what types of activities you need outfits for and how often. That way you can focus on closing any gaps in your wardrobe during the overhaul, and, at the same time, avoid adding to already jam-packed areas.

A five-step lifestyle analysis

 Work your way through these five steps to map out your lifestyle and wardrobe needs.

STEP 1

Write a list of every activity you do in an average two weeks. Include everything from lounging at home to meeting clients for dinner at fancy restaurants. For pointers, refer to the outfits you tracked in chapter 2. On your list, include an estimate of how many days out of two weeks you typically need an outfit for each activity, like the example below.

- Work (office): 7
- Work (from home): 2
- Presenting at a conference: 1
- Date night: 3
- Gym: 3
- Hiking: 1
- Going out at night: 2
- Chilling at home: 6
- Black-tie events: 1
- Meeting friends (daytime): 4

STEP 2

Create categories of activities for which you can wear the same type of outfits and add up the number of times you'll need an outfit for each category. Think daytime, nightlife, work, special occasions, working out, and so on. For example, since I work from home, I wear roughly the same type of clothes on a lazy Sunday afternoon and on a regular weekday when I'm not meeting anyone, so I can just group both of these under "Casual daytime stuff."

- Work (corporate dress code, for working at the office and conferences): 8
- Daytime (working from home, meeting up with friends): 6
- Semifancy (date night and going out at night): 5
- Chilling at home: 6
- Black-tie: 1
- Working out (gym and hiking): 4

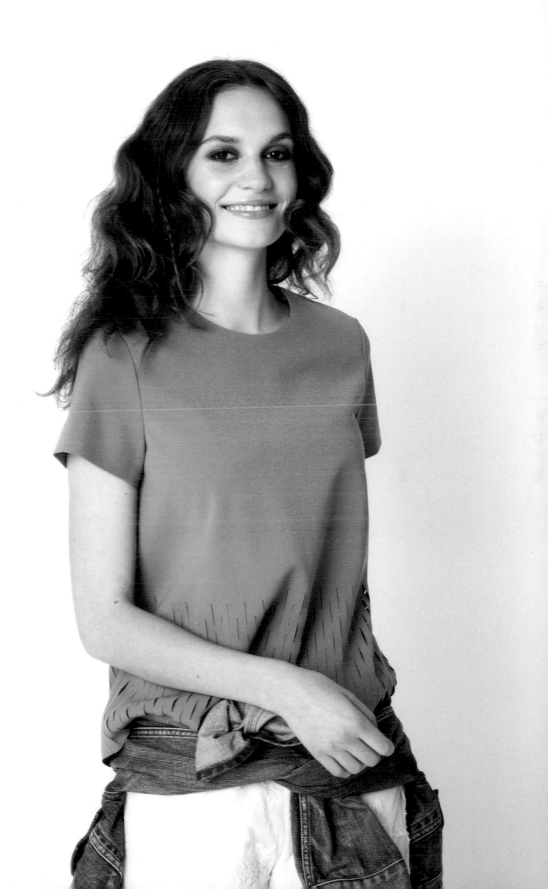

STEP 3

Now comes the fun part. Draw a pie chart that represents how often you need an outfit in an average two weeks for each of your categories. Don't worry about exact measurements; you are just trying to visualize the proportions, so eyeballing is fine.

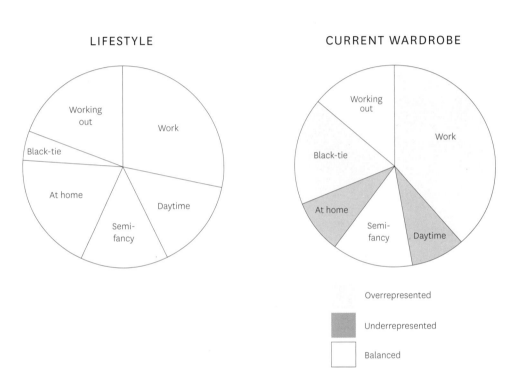

LIFESTYLE

CURRENT WARDROBE

Overrepresented

Underrepresented

Balanced

STEP 4

Draw another pie chart, but this time one that represents your current wardrobe (using the same activity categories as segments). Now, compare your two pie charts. Which categories are under-, over-, or well-represented?

STEP 5

Building a great wardrobe is not just about making sure you have *enough* clothes for whatever you want to do; each individual piece in your wardrobe should also be functional and work well for whatever activity you're dressing for.

For example, if you work in an office that's heavily air-conditioned year-round and you are always freezing, stock your wardrobe with a range of knits, heavyweight blazers, and tights instead of open-toed shoes and sleeveless blouses. Similarly, if you are on your feet all day, skip the five-inch heels and make sure you have a few chic but comfy boots or lower-heeled options to choose from.

And sure, all this is common sense. You know you should pick clothes that you feel comfortable in and that work with your day-to-day life. But sometimes, and especially when you are standing in a crammed changing room, it can be hard to remember everything. My advice: Write yourself a little list so you have something to refer back to the next time you are out shopping.

Here's how. Go through your activity categories one by one and, for each, ask yourself this: ideally, what specific functional criteria do you want a piece for that category to fulfill. Use the questions below as a starting point:

- What weather condition and general temperature should a piece from this category be tailored to? What is the climate like where you live? Will you be indoors or outdoors? Do you get hot or cold easily?
- Does a piece from this category need to conform to a special dress code? Think standard business attire, smart casual, covering tattoos or piercings, black-tie, white-tie, and so on.
- For shoes, how much walking will you be doing? What heel height do you prefer?
- For bags, what type of things will you be carrying with this piece? What size, weight, and internal structure would be ideal?
- For all your clothes, to what level of maintenance are you prepared to commit? If a weekly trip to the dry cleaner does not fit into your budget or busy schedule, don't buy anything that you can't just throw in the wash. If you are not a fan of ironing, stock your wardrobe with pieces made from fabrics that either don't wrinkle easily or don't need to be super crisp to look good (such as linen). Figure out how much time you can put into caring for your clothes and then find clothes that fit into that limit.

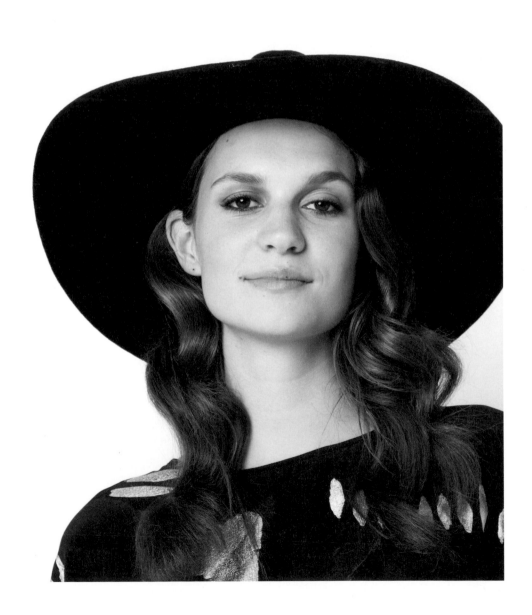

Setting priorities

Once you're ready to overhaul your wardrobe (see chapter 13 for a complete guide), aim to restock *underrepresented* areas first, whether that is your work wear, daytime clothes, or gym gear. For example, if you discovered you have plenty of clothes for all the special occasions in your life but not nearly enough for the day-to-day stuff that you spend 90 percent of your time doing, make it a point to use the first chunk of your budget to close that gap.

And unless your closet is bursting at the seams, don't worry about downsizing *overrepresented* areas just yet. As long as you love every single piece, more options are rarely a problem. Just make a mental note to hold off on buying any more stuff for that area for a while, and put that money toward restocking underrepresented areas instead.

09/ Closet composition 101

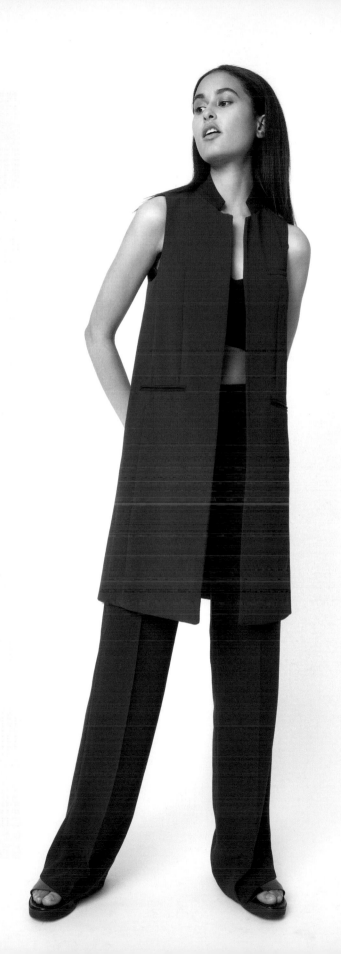

Following is a blueprint for building a fully functional
wardrobe that expresses your style, is easy to mix and
match, and gives you plenty of outfit options along
the entire spectrum of super casual to super fancy.

When I was younger, I bought clothes haphazardly. I had no strategy whatsoever.
Every single thing in my closet was something I had picked up here or there
because it looked cute on the rack. I rarely thought about how that candy-colored
sweater or A-line skirt might fit in with the rest of my wardrobe and what other
pieces I could wear it with. I liked it and so I bought it. Here's what I know now:
your wardrobe should be more than just a collection of stand-alone pieces.

A great wardrobe is like a well-oiled machine that
consists of interrelated parts that all work together,
allowing you to mix and match freely and create a ton
of different outfits that all suit your personal style.

But how do you build a wardrobe like that? You need a good strategy, a blueprint.
In this chapter, I'll show you one of three such strategies that you can use to
map out your ideal wardrobe. We'll talk about the other two strategies, which
are based on color palettes and outfit formulas, in chapters 10 and 11.

It's all about balance

The idea of strategy number one is to make sure your closet contains a
balanced mix of three types of items:

1. Key pieces that really signify the essence of your style and that you can wear
   in lots of different ways
2. Statement pieces that add variety to your looks and help you express
   different facets of your style

3. Basics that balance out bolder pieces and give the rest of your pieces a neutral backdrop

Working with a threefold structure like this has lots of benefits:

- It is a fail-proof way to ensure that every new piece you buy fulfills a clear role and will fit into the larger framework of your wardrobe.
- It helps you curate a balanced closet by preventing you from buying only statement pieces or blowing your entire budget on six versions of the same T-shirt.
- It's a fast track to making sure your wardrobe contains plenty of outfit options for any mood or occasion and is well balanced along the entire spectrum from dressed down to dressed up. Do you need an outfit for a super-fancy dinner party? Build an outfit that consists solely of statement pieces. Do you want to look casual but polished? Wear a couple of key pieces with basic shoes. Want to wear a statement top and your favorite heels during the day? Pair them with basic pants and minimal accessories. Easy peasy.

What makes a basic a basic?

A white button-down, jeans, a plain T-shirt: All are typical basics, right? Not so fast! Contrary to what fashion magazines may have led you to believe, there is no single definition of what makes something a basic, a key piece, or a statement piece. It all depends on your personal style. My own style leans more toward the casual side, and so, for me, things like large-scale patterns or shoes with a heel higher than two inches are typically statement pieces. But for someone with a bolder style those same items might be key pieces or even basics. All that matters is the relationship between the three functions in your wardrobe: basics are more casual than key pieces, and key pieces are more casual than statement pieces.

Next, we'll look at each type of wardrobe essential in more detail to help you find the right key pieces, statement pieces, and basics for your personal style.

Key Pieces

Your key pieces are the workhorses of your wardrobe. They reflect the look and feel of your personal style 100 percent and are ultra versatile and optimally tailored to your lifestyle. The perfect key pieces for your style are neither particularly bold nor plain but smack-dab in the middle of what you consider dressed up versus dressed down.

TYPICAL KEY PIECES

Jackets and outerwear; pants; skirts; shoes; bags; versatile tops

BUDGETING STRATEGY

Key pieces should get priority treatment during wardrobe revamps, because they will have the biggest impact on your ability to express your style. So buy them first and don't skimp on quality. Your key pieces should be as durable and well-constructed as possible to last you several years even with regular wear.

 With your style profile and mood board in front of you, ask yourself: Which five to ten concrete pieces best signify that style? Which key pieces do you need to be able to create outfits that represent that style?

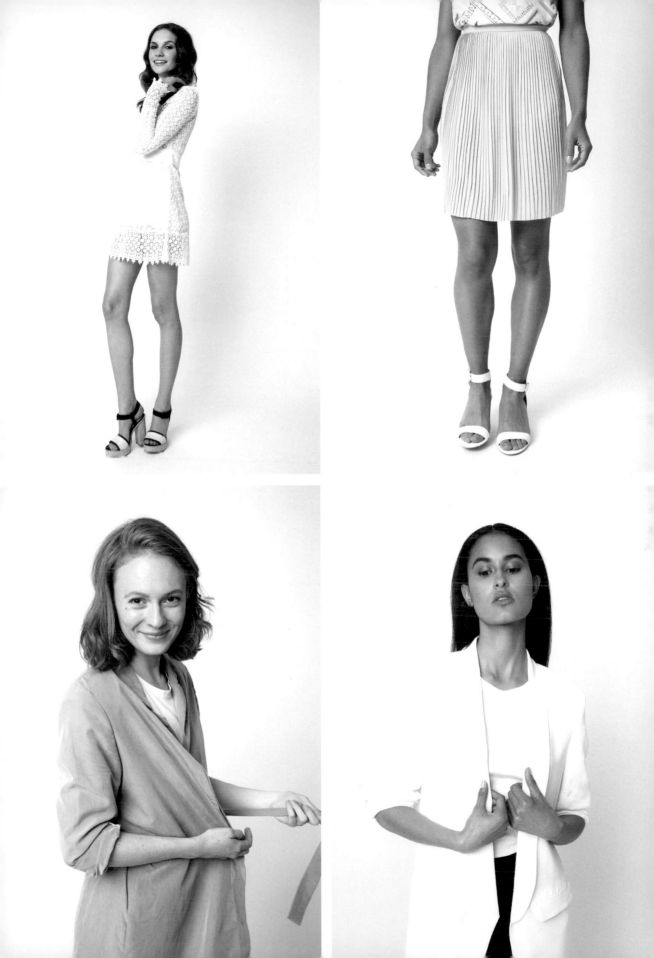

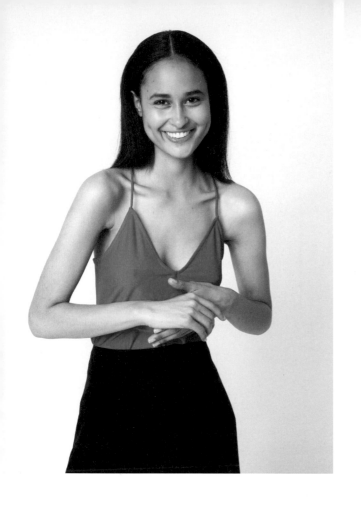

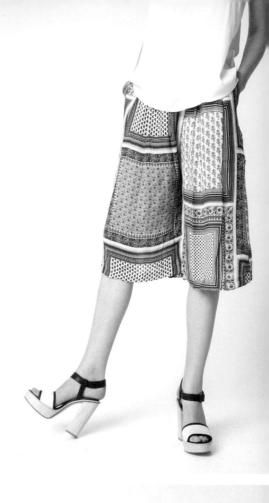

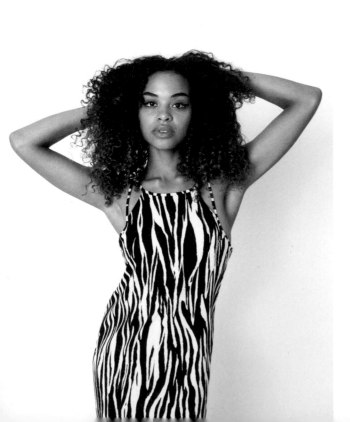

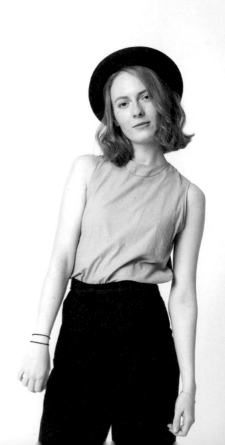

Statement Pieces

Statement pieces add variety to your wardrobe and give you a chance to express different aspects of your style. Wear them on their own for special occasions or whenever you feel like rocking a bolder look. Or pair them with your basics and key pieces for a little extra oomph.

Statement pieces don't have to be quite as mixable as the rest of your wardrobe, but as a rule of thumb, each piece should still work as part of at least three different outfits.

TYPICAL STATEMENT PIECES

Bold shoes, jewelry, and other accessories; tops, dresses, pants, and skirts in bolder colors or with unique details

BUDGETING STRATEGY

Since you'll likely get the least amount of wear out of your statement pieces, don't spend more on them than necessary. You want your pieces to look great and fit well, sure, but they don't necessarily have to last you more than a couple of years. Save your money for your key pieces instead.

 Identify any aspects in your style profile and mood board that are not yet covered by the five to ten key pieces you chose during the last exercise. Think colors, silhouettes, patterns, and so on. Based on these, choose five statement pieces.

Basics

Your basics' job is to support and balance out the rest of your pieces. They can tone down a bold look and give other pieces a neutral foundation to stand on. And they can also be used to fill in any gaps (for example, when you know your statement dress will run the show for the night but you still need a pair of shoes to wear).

Read more about the importance of paying attention to details when shopping for basics on page 200.

Your basics should be simpler than your key and statement pieces in terms of color, cuts, and details. But *simple* doesn't mean boring or cookie-cutter. Every piece in your wardrobe should reflect your style, and that includes your basics.

TYPICAL BASIC PIECES

Tops; T-shirts; jeans; and plain pants, skirts, and shoes

BUDGETING STRATEGY

Since your basics will likely be less structured and detailed than your other pieces, you should be able to find high-quality versions at all price points. An exception here are more structured pieces like blazers or jeans, which depend on an exact fit.

 Imagine you owned the five to ten key pieces and the five statement pieces you selected during the previous exercises, but nothing else. Brainstorm a few outfits you could build for different occasions. Which five to ten basics would you need to complete your mini wardrobe?

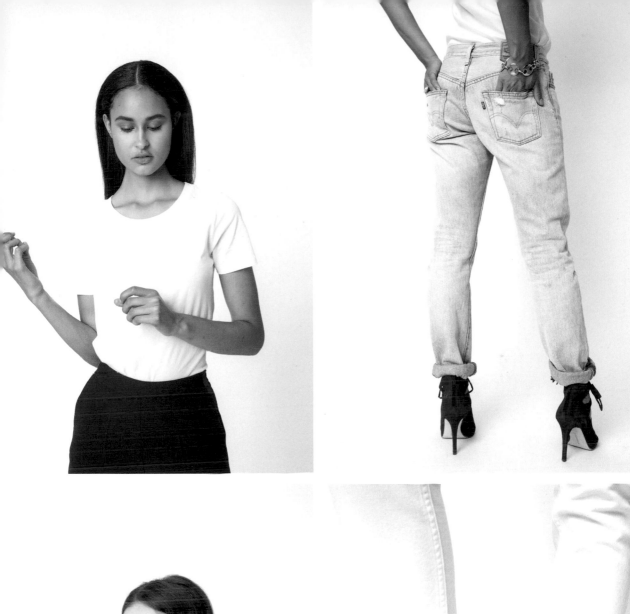

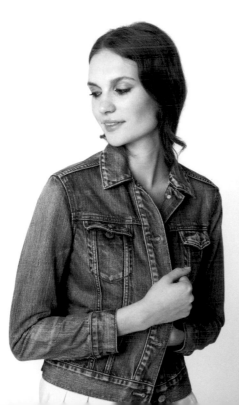

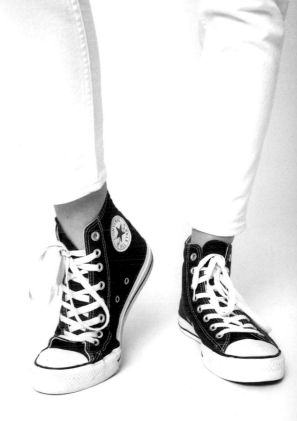

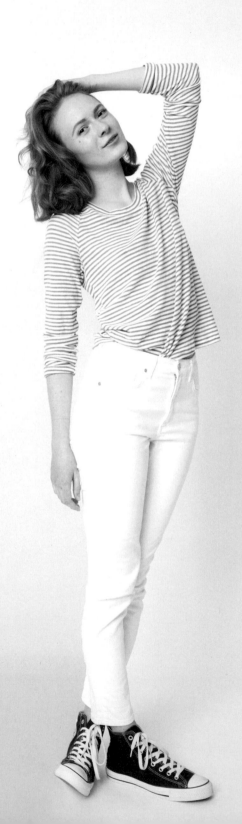

Assessing your current wardrobe

The point of the three thought experiments in this chapter was to help you come up with a mini wardrobe that's perfectly balanced and tailored to your personal style—regardless of what's currently sitting in your closet. Keep that mini wardrobe in your style file for now: you'll use it later on, alongside all your ideas from other chapters, to create a concrete shopping list for your wardrobe overhaul in chapter 13.

> A thought experiment is a creativity technique that makes it easier to come up with fresh new ideas by removing all outside restrictions and working off of a blank slate.

Complete these two last steps to figure out how much overlap there is between your ideal mini wardrobe and your current closet.

STEP 1

How balanced is your current wardrobe? Does it contain a good mix of key pieces, basics, and statement pieces? Or too little of one, not enough of the other?

STEP 2

Go back over the list of key pieces, basics, and statement pieces that you made during the last few exercises and compare it to your current wardrobe. Cross out any items that you already own (or a similar version of it).

10 / Selecting a versatile color palette

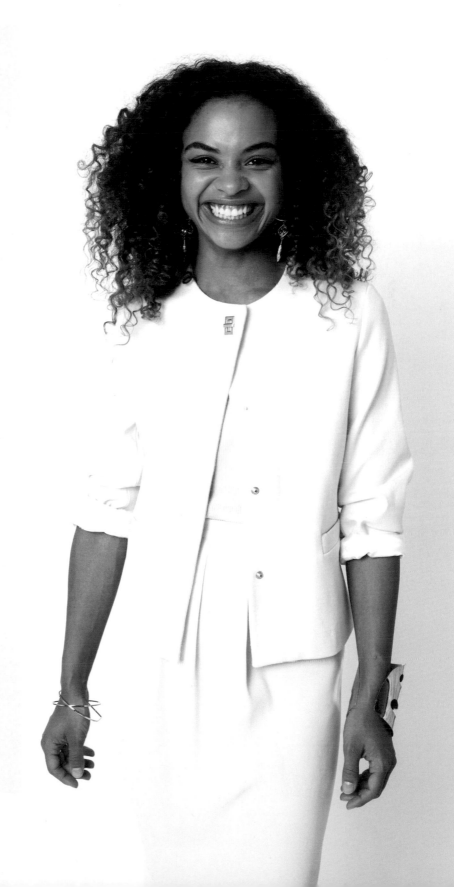

Color lovers unite! Learn all about the ins and outs of color palettes and how to create your own from scratch. Twelve sample color palettes are included to get you started.

Whether you like to dress in all colors of the rainbow, prefer a chic monochrome look, or favor something in between, your color likes and dislikes are one of the most important components of your personal style.

Color has the power to instantly trigger a mood, an emotion, or an association to a culture or an era. For example, most of us associate pastel shades with youth and innocence, silvers and blues with calmness and sophistication, and deep purples and reds with power and status.

Many of these associations with colors are universal to an extent, and some are cultural, but our personal life story also shapes these associations and provides each one of us with a very unique preference for certain colors.

The easiest way to make sure your wardrobe reflects that preference is to create your own color palette.

Building a color palette is the second of three strategies that works great for mapping out your ideal wardrobe. It is a super fun exercise that gives you a concrete blueprint you can use to curate a cohesive wardrobe that's easy to mix and match. Your color palette will also help you out when it comes to putting together outfits that are 100 percent in tune with your style. Plus, once you have tailored your closet to your color palette, shopping for new pieces is as easy as pie—that new sweater or pair of boots will not only fit straight in with the rest of your clothes, you'll also have lots and lots of pieces to wear it with.

Color palettes 101

What makes a great color palette? A few things: Your color palette should consist of six to twelve colors that work well with each other and reflect your style. On top of that, each color in your palette should have a clear function, depending on the role you want it to play in your wardrobe.

MAIN COLORS

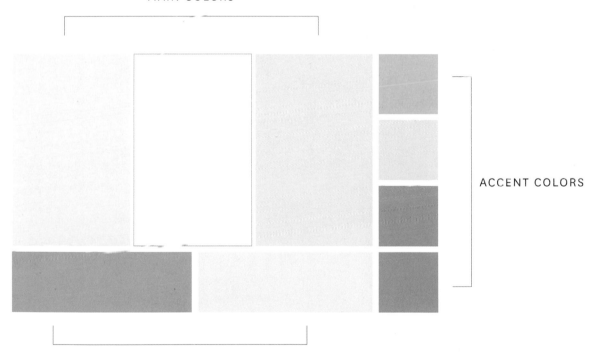

ACCENT COLORS

NEUTRAL COLORS

MAIN COLORS

The main colors in your palette should reflect the essence of your style concept and really signify the overall look you are going for. If you're going for a classic seventies boho look, your main colors could be tan, carrot orange, and mustard yellow. If your style is a mix of gothic and punk elements, your main colors might be black and red. If you're going for an Elle Woods in *Legally Blonde* look, your main colors are hot pink, magenta, and violet.

Your main colors are the equivalent of your favorite *style* colors. What colors do you love to wear? Which colors aren't you wearing yet that you want to play a major role in your wardrobe?

Any color of the rainbow, from a mousy gray to fuchsia pink, could be a main color depending on your specific style, so feel free to pick whichever colors you think best reflect the profile you created for your style. The only caveat is that all main colors should be ones that you can see yourself wearing a lot and that you feel super comfortable in. If your style profile is really bold and you have no problem wearing a lot of bright red, tangerine, and turquoise, go ahead and include those as your main colors. If not, simply reserve brighter colors like that for your accent shades or consider using a more muted version (perhaps a soft salmon or slate green).

ACCENT COLORS

Your accent shades add variety to your look and give you a chance to explore different facets of your style. Accent shades should work especially well for statement pieces and accessories that you would pair with your main colors and neutrals.

For example, two of my very favorite colors are light pink and apricot. I rarely want to dress in either of these colors head-to-toe (although I have on occasion). I prefer wearing them in small doses. I own a gorgeous light pink knit sweater as well as some pink and apricot scarves, purses, and tops. Whenever I wear these pieces, they are the focus point of my outfit and so I make sure to pair them with either a neutral (like light-wash denim jeans) or a piece in one of my main colors (white or sand) to give them a blank canvas.

For maximum mix-and-match potential, try to choose accent colors that work with each neutral and at least two of your main colors (bonus points if they go with each other as well).

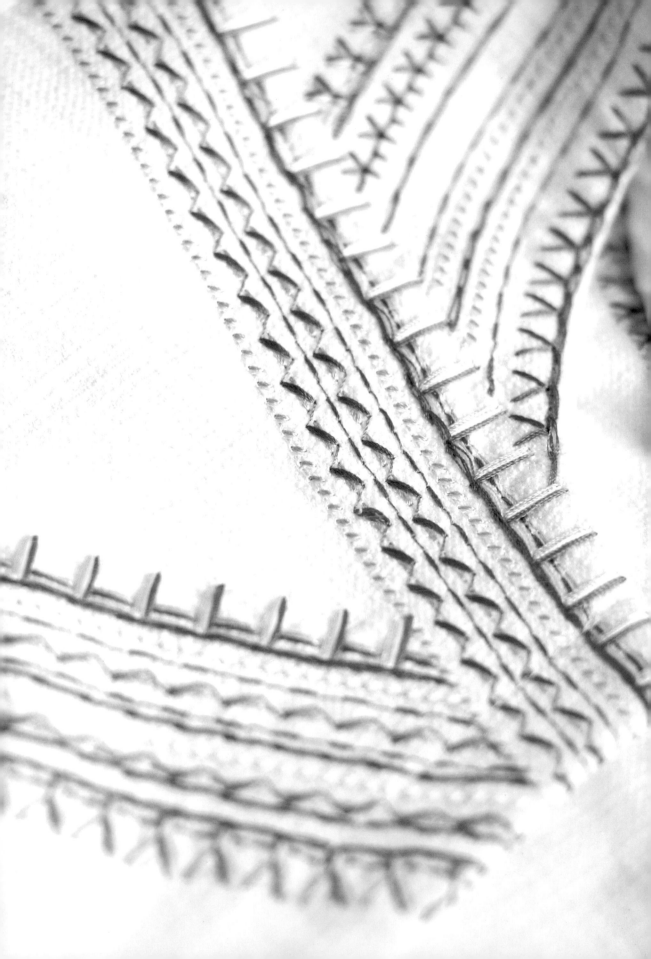

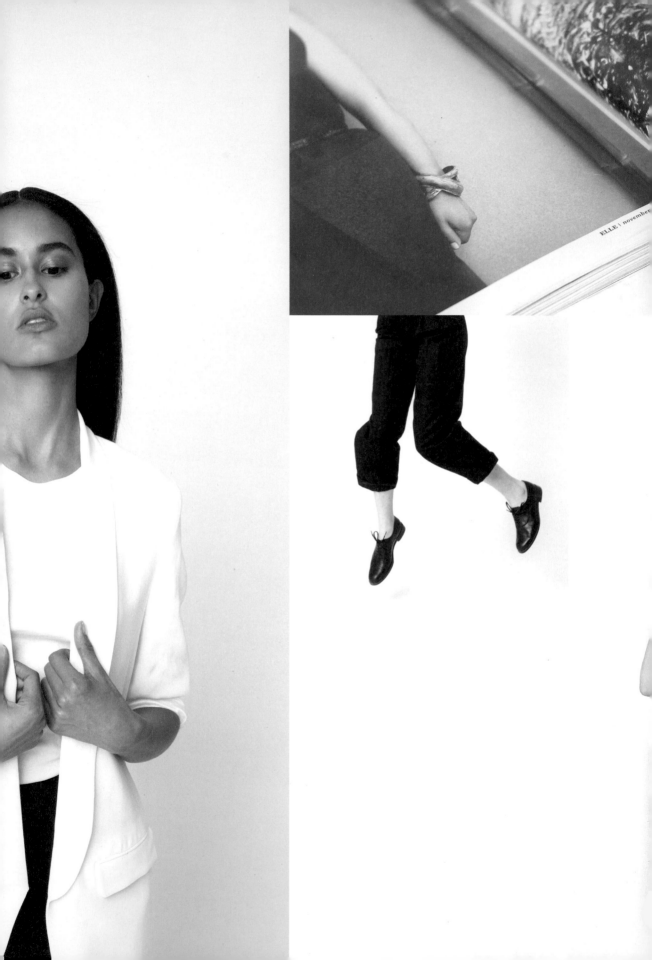

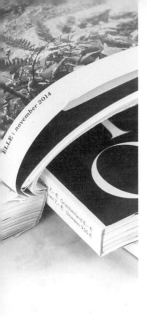

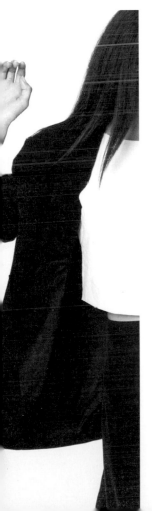

NEUTRAL COLORS

The neutral shades in your color palette are there to support and balance out the other colors.

For example, if you want to wear your pistachio green shift dress, you know that will be running the show and so you pair it with some simple white pumps in order to not overpower your look. Or if you want to wear a sapphire blue top during the day, you might wear it with a more neutral pair of pants, like your favorite pair of jeans, to tone it down.

Obvious choices for neutrals are white, black, gray, navy, and sand, and all washes of denim.

But in general, it's a good idea to pick your neutral shades only *after* you have chosen your main and accent colors. That way you will be able to see the overall theme of your palette and can select complimentary neutrals that will go well with every other shade. For example, if your palette includes several shades of green, a tomato red, and orange, you could make tan or another warm brown one of your neutrals, to complement the overall warm tone of your palette. Or, if you've built a cool palette of pastel blues and purples, go with a medium-wash denim and heather gray.

If one or two of your main colors are a typical neutral shade like black or gray, those pieces can function as double-duty pieces and you don't necessarily need to choose separate neutral shades, although you can if you like. It's all about *how* you want to wear those colors. In my current color palette, two of my main colors (sand and white) can double up as neutrals and I wear those pieces both ways. For example, during the summer I often wear all white outfits, but I also use white T-shirts or white denim to balance out brighter colors. On the other hand, light-wash denim is strictly a neutral for me, because I wear those pieces only to tone down or fill in, never as the main attraction.

The relationship between color palettes and key pieces, basics, and statement pieces

Although the three functions of the colors in your palette overlap somewhat with the three types of items we talked about in chapter 9, they are not the same! You can have key pieces in neutrals or accent shades in addition to main colors, and you can have basic pieces in neutrals, main colors, and even accent shades.

Here's why: color is only *one* of the factors that determine what role a piece could play within the framework of your wardrobe. The silhouette, material, and details of the piece are just as important. A dress in a neutral shade (like black) might well be a statement piece for you because it's formfitting, embellished, or has other characteristics that put it into dressed-up territory.

Are you ready to build your own color palette?

To select colors for your palette, start by going back over your style profile and mood board and write a big list of colors that reflect your style. Then, look through your current closet. Which colors are you already wearing and loving? Add these to your list as well.

Next comes the tricky part: Pick your favorites and organize them into a palette, complete with main colors, neutrals, and accent shades. Play around with a few different constellations until you've found one that's wearable, versatile, and represents your personal style to a tee.

As you choose your colors, ask yourself these questions:

- How big of a role do I want this color to play?
- How do I want to wear this color—as the main focus of the outfit, a canvas for other colors, or as smaller accents?
- Does this color make me feel confident?
- Does this color go well with the other shades in the palette?

HOW MANY COLORS SHOULD I CHOOSE FOR MY PALETTE?

I generally recommend aiming for nine shades in total (three main colors, four accent shades, and two neutrals), but you can of course tweak these numbers however you want. For example, if your entire look is minimalist and monochrome, you may need no more than two main colors, one neutral, and three accent shades. On the other hand, if you like a lot of variety, you could include up to twelve shades, but don't go too crazy! Remember: Just because you didn't include a color in your palette doesn't mean you can't wear it ever again. Your color palette is only supposed to be a guide for helping you build a more cohesive wardrobe. So keep it simple and focus on colors that are truly essential to your style.

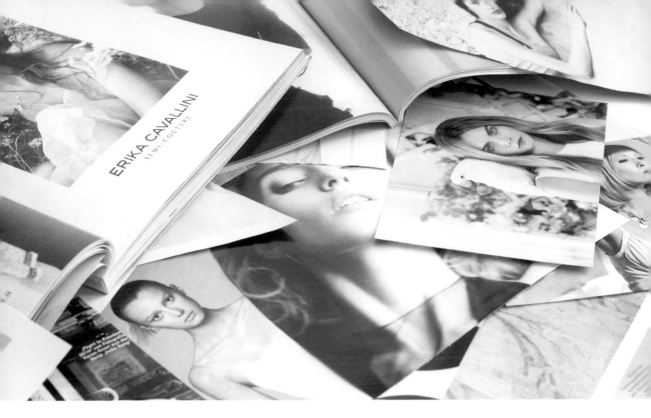

How to use your color palette

TO REBUILD YOUR WARDROBE FROM SCRATCH

You can use your color palette like a blueprint to build up a wardrobe that not only reflects your style but is also super mixable. Here's a quick preview of that process (you'll learn all about how to overhaul your wardrobe in chapter 13): First, you need to identify which colors are still missing from your current wardrobe and to what extent (there's an exercise on page 135 to help you do just that). Then, when it comes to writing a shopping list for your wardrobe overhaul, you can specify roughly how many pieces you still need in each color and what your priorities are. Always prioritize main colors, because they will have the biggest impact on how well you can express your style.

TO MAKE SURE NEW PIECES FIT INTO YOUR WARDROBE

Once you have built up a core set of pieces that reflects your color palette, you can start using your palette more like a rough guideline while you are out shopping. There's no need to wear exclusively the colors from your palette, but make sure that each new piece at least works with several of the colors in your palette so you know you'll have something to wear it with.

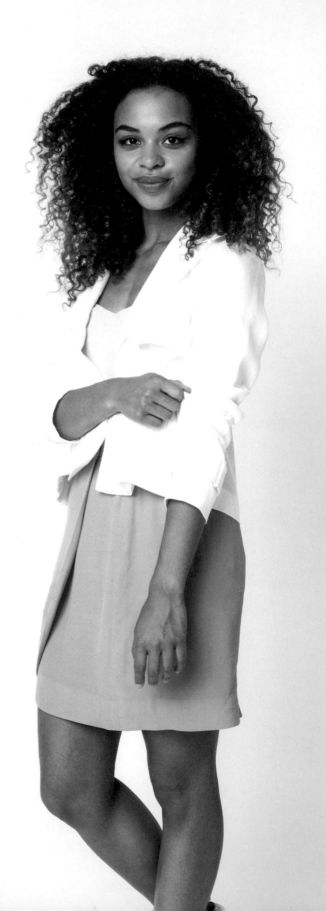

Next steps: Tailoring your current wardrobe to your color palette

 Once you have selected a versatile color palette, compare it to the clothes that are currently in your closet. How many pieces of each color do you already own? Add a quick note about your findings to your style file, like this:

I already own plenty of pieces that fit two of my main colors: black and navy blue, but none whatsoever that come close to my third main color (teal). I'm also relatively set in terms of my two neutrals (dark-wash denim and charcoal). For accent colors, I own a couple of lavender pieces, but not enough. My other three accent shades (mint, red, and a lighter blue) are nonexistent. In summary: I need a lot of pieces in teal, a few more in each of my three missing accent shades, and perhaps one or two additional lavender pieces.

You'll use your note to write a shopping list for your wardrobe overhaul later on page 161.

In the picture on the left, Lucia is wearing two of her main colors, peach and light blue, with some neutral white basics.

Sample Color Palettes

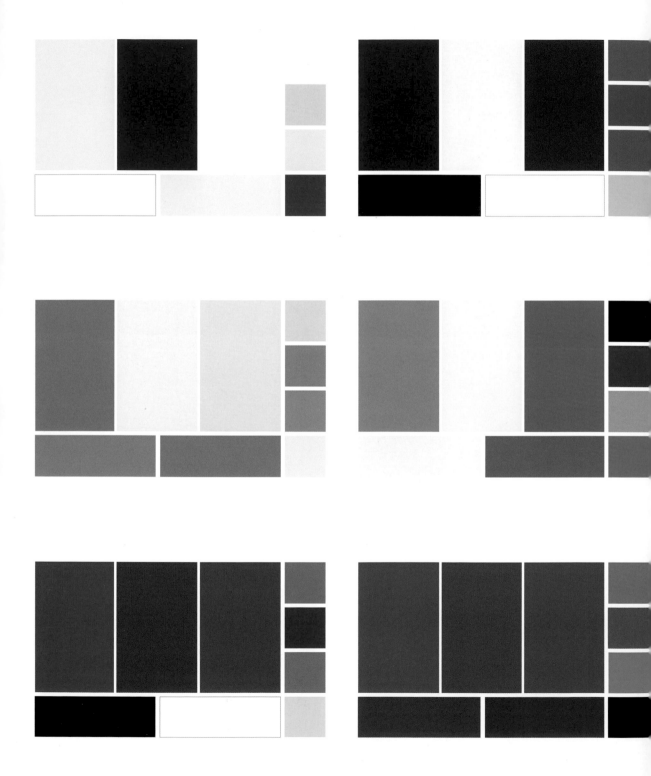

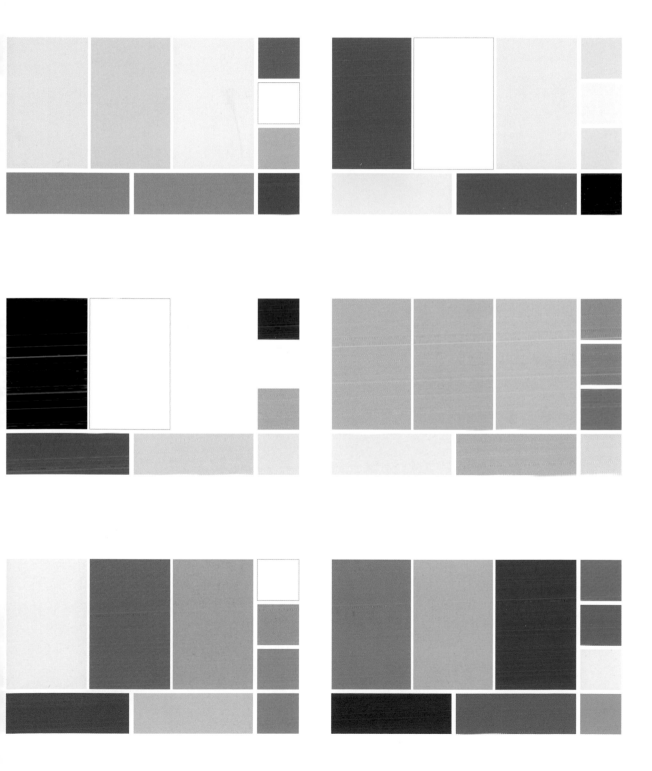

11 / Working with outfit formulas

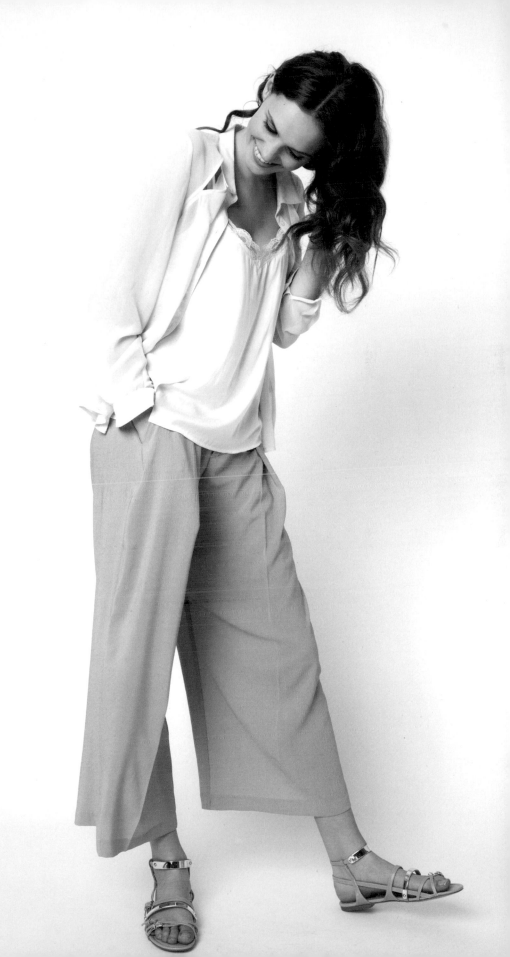

Take your wardrobe to the next level and streamline your morning routine! Plus, learn the secret to making sure you never again have *nothing* to wear.

Working with outfit formulas is one of my favorite techniques for building a mixable, versatile wardrobe (and the third strategy that you can use to map out your ideal closet).

What's an outfit formula? It's a *recipe* for a specific combination of items that you can wear in lots of different versions. If you like, you can also wear an outfit formula like a *uniform*, with very little variation. If you're into the idea of having a set uniform, you're in good company—some of the biggest style icons of our time wear a version of their uniform over and over again, from US *Vogue* editor in chief Anna Wintour (sunglasses, a patterned knee-length dress, heels, and a chunky necklace) to fashion designer Karl Lagerfeld (slim-fitting black slacks, a black blazer, a white shirt with a high collar, a tie, and gloves). Here are some examples:

- Flared jeans + simple camisole + cardigan + flat sandals
- Pencil skirt + knit sweater + blazer + heels

The idea is that you choose a few outfit formulas that reflect your style and which you feel confident wearing and then curate several different pieces that you can mix and match for each *ingredient* of your outfit formulas. For example, if one of your outfit formulas is *A-line mini skirt + button-down shirt + slip-on mules*, you could stock your wardrobe with two A-line skirts, three button-down shirts, and two pairs of mules, all in different but mixable colors, patterns, and materials.

That's only seven pieces in total—but those seven pieces give you twelve different outfit combinations to choose from! And that's only for one single outfit formula. Imagine if you had three outfit formulas hanging in your closet. Not only would you have three times twelve distinct outfits to choose from,

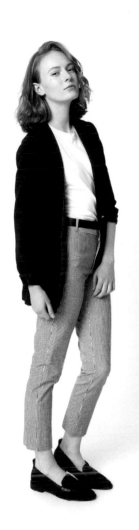

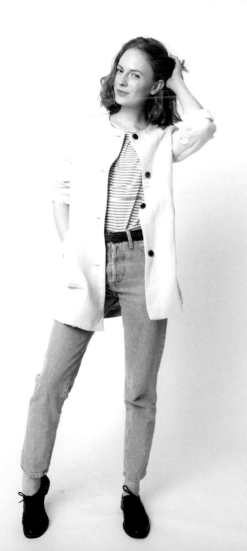

you could also mix them all with each other, style them up with accessories . . . *et voilà*: you've got a wardrobe that's packed with different outfit options that all fit your style.

Of course, not everything in your closet needs to be a part of one of your formulas. Think of your outfit formula as your *style staples*. You can wear them as per recipe but you can also modify them and mix them with the rest of your wardrobe, perhaps add an extra layer like a jacket, and then top everything off with accessories, hair, and makeup.

How to select outfit formulas for your style

 Complete these next three steps in your style file!

STEP 1: LOOK AT WHAT OUTFIT FORMULAS YOU ARE ALREADY WEARING

Even if you hadn't heard of the concept before, it's likely that you already have at least one or two outfit formulas in rotation at the moment. Do you tend to wear some type of slacks or chinos with a looser-fitting shirt and ballet flats for work? That's an outfit formula right there! And your go-to mini dress + ankle boots + coat combo? That's another one!

Go back over the two weeks' worth of outfits you documented for chapter 2 and list every combination that comes up at least three times. Then take a moment to think about why you keep wearing each particular formula and cross out any that you are not wearing for a good reason. Good reasons would be that it makes you feel confident, it's super comfortable, or you simply love the look of it. Repeatedly wearing a formula because you are stuck in a rut, want to cover up, or couldn't think of anything else to wear, however, would be bad reasons.

STEP 2: FIND OUTFIT FORMULAS THAT REFLECT YOUR IDEAL STYLE

Just like every other aspect of your wardrobe, your outfit formulas should above all reflect your personal style. So once you've made a list of all the outfit formulas you are already wearing, take a few minutes to look through your style profile and mood board and figure out which outfit formulas would best reflect the overall look you want to go for. Essentially, an outfit formula is a specific combination of silhouettes, so pay special attention to any inspiration you collected on cuts and silhouettes and also all information you gathered during your fieldwork stage about how you like things to fit. Add your favorites to the list of outfit formulas you are already wearing and liking.

STEP 3: CHOOSE YOUR FAVORITE OUTFIT FORMULAS TO GET STARTED

From your list of contenders, choose the two to four outfit formulas that you (1) think best reflect your style in terms of the silhouettes you like and (2) would feel super comfortable and confident in. If you have to wear very different types of clothes for work, you could split these up and choose two formulas for work and two for evenings and weekends. For now, choose only your absolute favorites; you can always add more later if you need to.

Implementing your outfit formulas

To implement your outfit formulas, start by going through your closet and pick out anything that could work as an ingredient. Then, see where you stand and identify where your biggest gaps are.

As a general rule, it's a good idea to first make sure you have at least *two* versions for all formula ingredients. That way you can start wearing and mixing pieces within your formulas sooner rather than later. Once you've curated those two first pieces per ingredient, you can gradually add more if you want to, and as your budget allows.

When it comes to choosing pieces, aim for variety! If you need five tank tops, don't just grab a stack of basic ones in different shades of gray. One or two basics in neutral colors is fine, but make the other tank tops key or statement pieces and pick different necklines, patterns, and details. Your goal is to cover as big of a range within each little group of ingredients as possible. Using that approach will allow you to express many different facets of your personal style, even with a smaller number of pieces.

Time for another list! For each one of your chosen outfit formulas, write down a quick description of every piece you already own by ingredient. Next, think about how many pieces are still missing per ingredient and write down any first ideas about what type of pieces you may want to buy. All this information will come in handy once you are ready to overhaul your wardrobe in chapter 13 and are trying to decide what pieces to put on your shopping list.

Here are examples for a warm-weather climate.

OUTFIT FORMULA 1
Skinny jeans + tunic + flat sandals

OUTFIT FORMULA 2
Mini dress + oversize button-down
(tie at waist) + sneakers

SKINNY JEANS

Light-wash ankle-length jeans
White high-waisted jeans

TUNIC

Ivory tunic with lace detailing
Amber tunic with embroidery
Darker, patterned tunic

FLAT SANDALS

Tan suede leather sliders
Dark brown fringed sandals

MINI DRESS

Cream dress with floral pattern
Light gray dress with skater skirt
Tan suede dress with button front

OVERSIZE BUTTON-DOWN

Denim shirt
White lacy blouse
Another shirt in moss green or teal

SNEAKERS

White high-tops
Gray canvas low-tops

■ Missing pieces

Advanced wardrobe engineering: how to prevent laundry bottlenecks

Another reason I'm such a fan of the outfit formula concept is because it gives you a chance to optimize your wardrobe by avoiding laundry bottlenecks.

Outfit formulas and laundry ratios also come in handy for traveling. Simply pick one or two formulas, throw a couple of pieces for each into your suitcase, and you're all set.

Because here's the thing: the reason we usually run out of clothes is rarely because we literally have no clean clothes left, but because we are missing one single component, usually underwear or a top, or anything that needs a wash sooner than pieces like skirts or jackets.

The easy solution: Make sure you have *more* of those pieces in your closet. And, if you want to be precise, use outfit formulas that give you all the information you need to calculate exactly *how many* more!

Let's say one of your outfit formulas is *jeans + T-shirt + cardigan*, just to keep it really simple. For each formula ingredient, figure out how many times you can usually wear a piece before it needs to be washed.

For example:
T shirts: 1 times
Jeans: 4 times
Cardigan: 4 times

This means that if you want to wear that outfit formula four times between laundry days, you could wear the same pair of jeans and the same cardigan but would need four T-shirts.

You don't have to get super precise with this, but it's a good idea to keep these laundry ratios in mind when it comes to stocking your wardrobe. The sooner a piece needs a wash, the more versions you need in your wardrobe, and vice versa.

Two-week sample outfit plan

To show you a concrete example of how outfit formulas can be used in action, here are two weeks' worth of outfits, all created from only two outfit formulas, each of which contains two or three pieces.

OUTFIT FORMULA 1
Knee-length skirt + knit sweater + coat + heels

OUTFIT FORMULA 2
Straight-leg pants + oversize shirt + jacket + flats

3 KNEE-LENGTH SKIRTS

Black leather skirt

Camel ribbed-knit pencil skirt

Navy A-line skirt with
jacquard pattern

3 KNIT SWEATERS

Burgundy cable knit

Champagne sequinned

Thin black turtleneck

2 COATS

Tan trench

Navy wool

2 PAIRS OF HEELS

Ruby-red pumps

Black 4-inch ankle boots

2 PAIRS OF STRAIGHT-LEG PANTS

Dark-wash jeans

Black cigarette pants

3 OVERSIZE SHIRTS

Burgundy-black check

Olive-green linen shirt

White silk shirt

2 JACKETS

Black oversize blazer

Khaki parka

2 PAIRS OF FLATS

Leopard print flats

Black lace-up flats

MONDAY

Navy A-line skirt with jaquard pattern

Thin black turtleneck

Tan trench coat

Black 4-inch ankle boots

TUESDAY

Black leather skirt

Burgundy cable knit sweater

Navy wool coat

Black 4-inch ankle boots

WEDNESDAY

Black cigarette pants

Burgundy-black check shirt

Black oversize blazer

Black lace-up flats

THURSDAY *Outfit formula mix!*

Camel ribbed-knit pencil skirt

Olive-green linen shirt

Tan trench coat

Leopard print flats

FRIDAY *Outfit formula mix!*

Dark-wash jeans

White silk shirt

Khaki parka

Ruby-red pumps

SATURDAY

Navy A-line skirt with jaquard pattern

Burgundy cable knit sweater

Navy wool coat

Black 4-inch ankle boots

SUNDAY *Outfit formula mix!*

Black leather skirt

Champagne sequinned sweater

Navy wool coat

Black lace-up flats

MONDAY

Black cigarette pants

Olive-green linen shirt

Khaki parka

Leopard print flats

TUESDAY *Outfit formula mix!*

Navy A-line skirt with jaquard pattern

White silk shirt

Black oversize blazer

Black lace-up flats

WEDNESDAY

Camel ribbed-knit pencil skirt

Thin black turtleneck

Tan trench coat

Black 4-inch ankle boots

THURSDAY

Dark-wash jeans

Burgundy-black check shirt

Khaki parka

Black lace-up flats

FRIDAY *Outfit formula mix!*

Black cigarette pants

Champagne sequinned sweater

Black oversize blazer

Ruby-red pumps

SATURDAY

Black leather skirt

Thin black turtleneck

Tan trench coat

Ruby-red pumps

SUNDAY

Dark-wash jeans

Olive-green linen shirt

Khaki parka

Leopard print flats

12 / Business hours: Tweaking your wardrobe for work

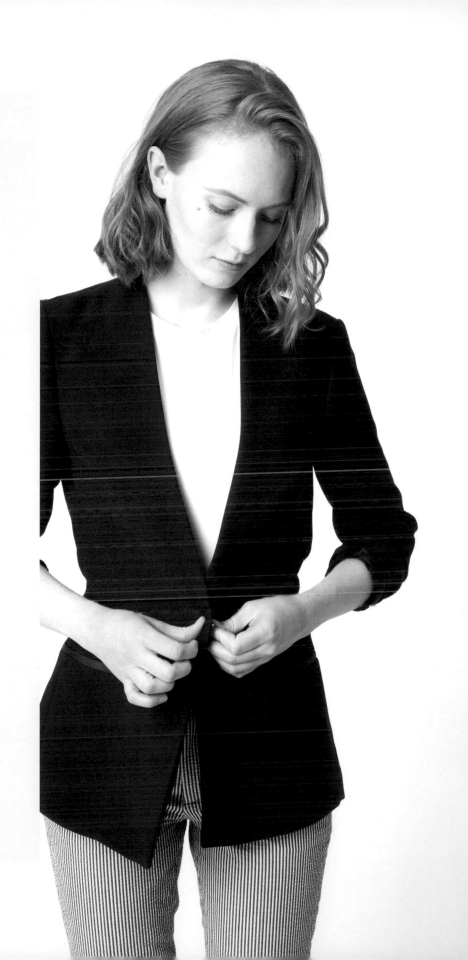

Curate a work wardrobe that makes you look and feel
professional, confident, and ready to tackle the day.

Whether you work at a corporate law firm, a tiny nonprofit, or from home,
having a great set of clothes to wear for work is important, not because of
how they make you look but because of how they make you feel.

If you have worked your way through the exercises in the last few chapters,
you probably have a pretty good idea of what you want your overall wardrobe
to look like by now. In this chapter, I'll show you a few additional tips and
techniques that you can use to optimize your closet for your work life.

Of course, your ideal business look depends in no small part on the dress code
of your work environment, so I've separated the advice into three sections:
corporate jobs, anywhere with a smart-casual dress code, and working from
home (as a student, freelancer, or business owner).

To get started, let's quickly go over some criteria that the ideal work wardrobe
should fulfill:

- It makes you look and feel professional and gives you confidence for
  presentations, meetings, or talks with the boss.
- It is 100 percent comfortable and functional, so you can concentrate on your
  work without having to worry about straps that dig in or a skirt that rides up.
- It should respect the company's dress code (spoken or unspoken) and
  culture yet still reflect your own personal style.

Corporate jobs

This includes jobs at most medium to large organizations, law firms, and
the financial industry. Your basic strategy will be to build a separate capsule
wardrobe that you wear solely for work (read more on capsule wardrobes
on page 172).

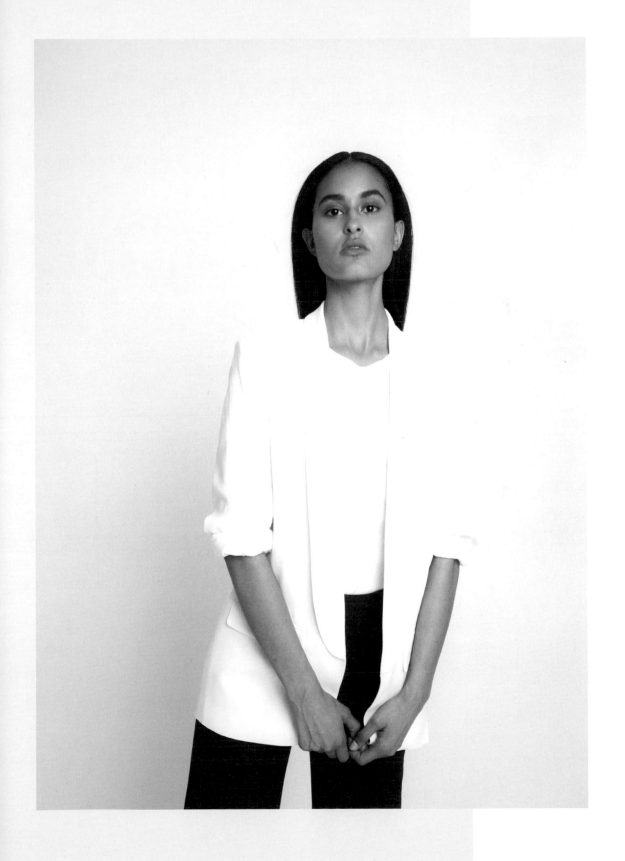

KEEP YOUR WORK WARDROBE SEPARATE FROM YOUR REGULAR WARDROBE

Regardless of your own personal style, if you work in an environment with a very strict professional dress code, I recommend you build a completely separate work wardrobe. A "dual wardrobe" model like this is not only way easier to plan but also means you can fully express your personal style in your free time and won't end up with a whole lot of stuff that's work-appropriate but only 50 percent your style.

CREATE A MINI STYLE PROFILE FOR YOUR WORK LOOK

As a guideline for your work capsule wardrobe, take some time to put together a separate mini style profile for your work wardrobe that reflects both your company's dress code *and* your style. If that seems like an impossible task, because to you, *corporate dress code* equals *drab and boring*, you might need to add a few new sources of inspiration to your list. As a first step, check out the other people in your office. What are they wearing, how do they interpret the dress code, and which details could you incorporate into your own look? If there aren't any stylish people in your office, expand your net! My favorite source for office-wear style inspiration is TV, where characters in shows are usually dressed in a way that's super chic but still realistic and therefore replicable. Once you have gathered some inspiration and decided on an overall work look, use the questions on page 87 to write your "business hours" mini style profile.

BUILD A WORK-ONLY CAPSULE WARDROBE

Once you have an overall idea of the kind of look you want to be able to create using your work wardrobe, focus on finding a few versatile, high-quality key pieces that could work as the framework of your wardrobe. Think tailored pants, skirts, a couple of blazers, and a few comfortable (!) pairs of shoes. Since your options are somewhat limited here in regard to the type of pieces you can choose, make it a point to get the details—fit, material, and color—right.

Instead of any old black blazer, aim to find one that fits your silhouette perfectly, consists of a high-quality fabric, and complements your shape. Next, find a range of tops in different styles (shirts, knit sweaters, cardigans) and colors that you can mix and match with your key pieces and that align well with your style. Your key pieces and tops make up your basic work-only capsule wardrobe, which is where you'll want to put the majority of your work-wear budget. You can then spruce up your work-only capsule wardrobe using accessories and statement pieces, some or all of which could come from your regular wardrobe. If chosen right, twenty pieces could be all you need (for example, three blazers, three pairs of pants, three skirts, eight tops, and three pairs of shoes).

PERSONALIZE WITH ACCESSORIES AND DETAILS

Accessories, single items, and smaller styling tweaks are the best ways to inject some personality into your office look without breaking the company's dress code. Go through your regular closet to look for pieces that could add some color or depth to your work outfits and tailor it a little more to your personal style with delicate jewelry, a statement necklace, a belt, glasses, a nice watch, nail polish, or a brighter top in one of your accent colors worn underneath a more neutral top. If you need more ideas, refer back to your workwear style profile and the inspiration you collected.

Smart-casual

This includes jobs at start-ups and smaller companies, and in creative industries and academia. Your basic strategy will be to curate a selection of more formal key pieces to pair with your regular clothes.

ANALYZE YOUR COWORKERS' STYLES

If you work in an environment without a dress code in the traditional sense, you obviously have a lot more freedom when it comes to your work attire. On the other hand, even when there isn't an official dress code, most companies will still have a handful of unspoken rules and guidelines that everyone follows. And these can be quite tricky to figure out if you're a newbie. So after your interview or on your first day, take a good look around to see what other people are wearing.

Is there literally no dress code at all, and people walk around in flip-flops and band T-shirts? Or does everyone seem to stick to the typical smart-casual look? Smart-casual essentially means no suits required, but you'll still want to look polished and avoid some basic office no-go items like strapless tops or dresses, halter tops or dresses, super low-cut tops, short shorts, and flip-flops.

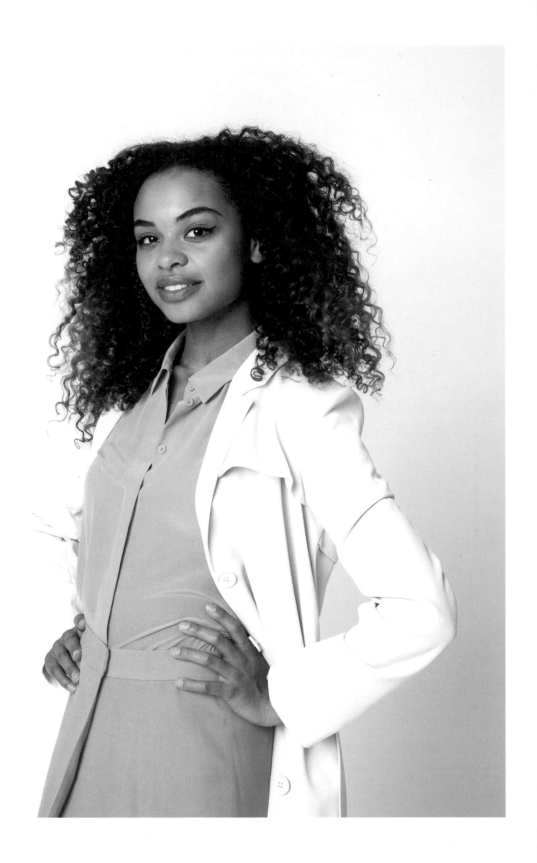

GO THROUGH YOUR WARDROBE

For people with full-time jobs in a smart-casual work environment, I generally recommend a three-section wardrobe structure:

- Section 1: Double-duty pieces you can wear for work and your personal life.
- Section 2: Free-time pieces that you can't wear for work, that are only for weekends and evenings.
- Section 3: More formal "add-on" pieces that you specifically buy for the job to pair with your pieces from section 1.

To set up your structure, go through your wardrobe and pick out everything that you could wear to work. This will likely include any basic tops, shirts, tailored pants, and skirts and dresses (in appropriate lengths, colors, and fabrics). Those pieces are your double-duty pieces that you can wear for evenings and weekends with the rest of your wardrobe and on their own or with more formal pieces for work.

BUY A COUPLE OF "ADD-ON" PIECES FOR WORK

Once you have identified your double-duty pieces, you need to analyze that pile and figure out what you might still need to buy to (1) fill any gaps and (2) add a few smarter options to your set. Always think in terms of the bigger groups: bottoms (pants, skirts, dresses), shoes, jackets, and tops. If your personal style is already relatively similar to "smart-casual," you might need nothing but perhaps another smart blazer, some oxfords, and a couple more nice shirts.

Even if the dress code at your company is smart-casual, it's a good idea to have at least one or two traditionally corporate outfits at hand for special events like a meeting with an investor or conferences. For example, you might want one blazer, a matching pair of pants or a skirt, some nice shoes, and one or two dressier shirts.

Working from home

This includes freelancers, students, and business owners. If you are the type of person that *doesn't* feel the need to change into something more comfortable as soon as they get home, you can skip this section, because you can just wear your regular wardrobe during the day. Everyone else: Consider adding some comfortable clothes to your wardrobe that make you feel put-together and ready for work.

ACKNOWLEDGE THAT YOUR WORK WARDROBE DESERVES ATTENTION

Yes, you can pretty much wear whatever all day long and hold client calls in your PJs—that's your total right as a student, freelancer, or business owner. But just because no one sees you doesn't mean your "work wardrobe" isn't important. If you go back up to the three criteria a good work wardrobe should fulfill, two of the three also apply to you: you want your clothes to make you feel confident and professional and you need them to be comfortable and functional.

On top of that, you want your clothes to put you in the right mindset for work. For me, getting to work is always a lot easier when I do what most people who have to commute to an office do: get up at a certain time, shower, get ready, get dressed, and sit at a desk that I use solely for work. Rituals like that are important because over time they essentially program your brain to go into work mode once you have done them. When you are your own boss, you need to create those rituals yourself, and your clothes can be a crucial part of that.

INVEST IN COMFORTABLE CLOTHES

Your work-from-home clothes don't have to be fancy, but they should make you feel polished and put together. Think comfy but nice T-shirts, long-line cardigans, comfortable pants, loose-fitting shirts, or whatever types of clothing you find the most comfortable that also reflect your style and makes you feel like *you*.

HAVE A COUPLE OF PROFESSIONAL OUTFITS AT HAND

Even if you work from home, you will likely have to leave the house from time to time for client meetings and work-related events, so make sure you have a few dressier outfits sitting in your closet for those occasions. Have a look through your calendar to get a feeling for how often you need a more professional look per month and then build up a small set of pieces that you can mix and match, perhaps a simple blazer, some heels, and a couple of nicer shirts.

After reading through this chapter, ask yourself: How happy are you with the clothes you currently wear to work? What changes do you want to make to your wardrobe? What additional pieces would help you optimize it for your professional life?

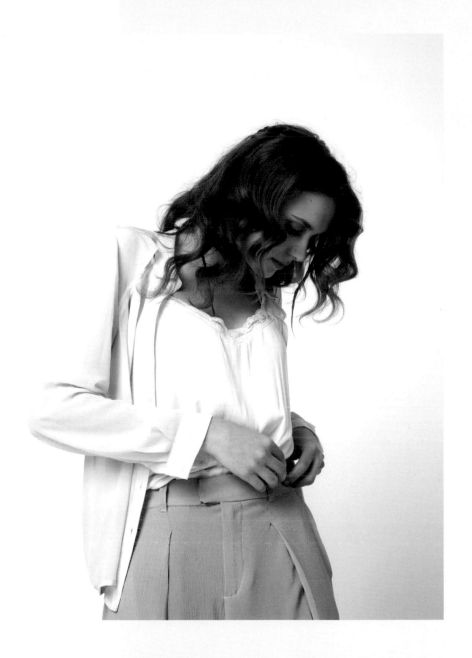

13 / Overhauling your wardrobe: A step-by-step road map

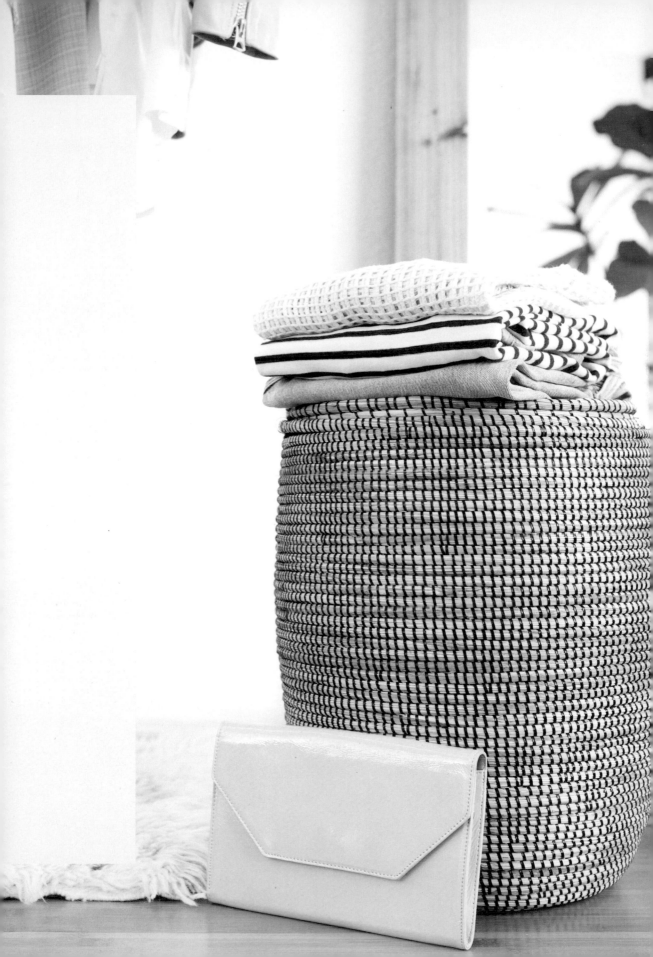

From a top-to-bottom revamp to a mini update, here's everything you need to know about overhauling your wardrobe, including how to turn your rough ideas into a concrete shopping list, what to buy first, and how to shop without getting overwhelmed.

Okay, so you've defined your personal style and mapped out your dream wardrobe. Now it's time to make that dream a reality! In this chapter, I'll walk you through the steps of overhauling your wardrobe and discuss the biggest do's and don'ts.

Spoiler alert! It all boils down to two things: take it slow and prioritize. In other words, don't buy everything at once! I know that's hard, especially when your current closet looks nothing like your dream wardrobe. But it's crucial. Building the perfect wardrobe (or even just a much-better-than-I-have-right-now wardrobe) is a long-term project. You need time to grow into your new style item by item and give yourself the chance to really think things through. And unless you have an unlimited budget (and who does?), you also simply need time to save up before you can buy everything you need at the level of quality you want.

But here's some good news: just because it will likely take you a while to build the perfect wardrobe doesn't mean you have to wait that long until you can start dressing according to your personal style. That's where the "prioritize" part comes in.

Some pieces in your dream wardrobe will have a bigger impact on your ability to express your style than others, for example, a great blazer that really signifies your style and that you can wear with everything, or a versatile pair of shoes in one of your main colors that also fills a glaring gap in your wardrobe. The trick is to identify these pieces and buy them first. That way, no matter your budget, every dollar you spend has the biggest possible immediate effect on your wardrobe.

The four-step overhaul

STEP 1: GET A COMPLETE OVERVIEW OF EVERYTHING YOU STILL NEED

If your wardrobe needs a big revamp, you may feel equally excited and overwhelmed right now—excited at the prospect of finally building a great wardrobe and overwhelmed because you know your wardrobe needs a ton of work and you don't know where to start.

The first step to combatting overwhelm is to get a complete overview of everything you still need to buy. So go through your style file and transfer all the notes from the last few chapters (about gaps in your wardrobe and ideas for pieces you could buy) to a new page, including the following information:

- The biggest gaps in your wardrobe (from chapter 7, Closet detox: The complete guide, page 92)
- Underrepresented areas in your lifestyle (from chapter 8, How to build a wardrobe that fits your real life (not your fantasy life), page 102)
- Missing key pieces, basics, and statement pieces (from chapter 9, Closet composition 101, page 112)
- Missing colors from your palette (from chapter 10, Selecting a versatile color palette, page 124)
- Pieces you need to create your outfit formulas (from chapter 11, Working with outfit formulas, page 138)
- Any additional pieces you need for work (from chapter 12, Business Hours. Tweaking your wardrobe for work, page 148)

STEP 2: TURN VAGUE IDEAS INTO CONCRETE PIECES

At this point your notes will likely include a mix of concrete pieces, like "burgundy pea coat," and vague descriptors, such as "clothes for casual Fridays" and "something in navy blue."

Your next goal is to turn as many of those vague descriptors into concrete pieces, so that you end up with a precise list of things to shop for.

For example, if your closet detox revealed a serious shortage of well-fitting pants, try to specify what type of pants would make a great addition to your wardrobe, in as much detail as possible and taking into account everything you have discovered about your style and dream wardrobe so far. Think color, materials, patterns, silhouettes, details, and also how many new pairs of pants you need.

And, whenever possible, see if you can come up with pieces that satisfy more than one quality on your list. For example, if your notes say "more clothes for work," "midi skirts," and "heather gray," one of your pieces could be a heather-gray midi skirt that's smart enough to wear for work. Or if you know you still need several casual tops that you can wear on the weekend as well as pieces in red, white, and black, add "casual red top," "casual black top," and "casual white top" to your list.

Streamline your list as you go along. For example, feel free to cross off "more blazers" if at a later stage you can specify that you want a "charcoal blazer" and a "navy blue blazer."

If you can't come up with a concrete piece for some points in your notes or can't decide whether you want that "light pink something" to be a top, dress, or pair of shoes, that's okay. Simply write "one additional piece in light pink (top, dress, or pair of shoes)" and move on.

STEP 3: ORGANIZE YOUR LIST BY PRIORITY

 To indicate priority, you can organize your pieces into groups (high, mid, and low priority, to keep it super simple) or rank them.

To organize your pieces, ask yourself the following:

1. How big of an impact will this piece have on my ability to create outfits that express my style? Prioritize pieces that really signify your personal style and that you can wear in lots of different ways:

- Key pieces (over basics and statement pieces)
- Pieces in main colors (over accent colors, neutrals, or colors that are not a part of your color palette)

- Pieces that are a part of one of your outfit formulas (over pieces that aren't)

2. How big is the gap that this piece would fill? Prioritize pieces that fill a big gap over pieces similar to what you already own:

- Pieces for activities and occasions that are currently underrepresented in your closet
- Pieces in colors that are missing from your wardrobe (over ones in a color already represented by a couple of items in your closet)
- Pieces for outfit formula ingredients you don't own, or have only one of (over pieces you already own a couple of)

What I need to buy

Here's an example of what your shopping list could look like once you've completed these three steps.

HIGH PRIORITY

long-line camel coat for winter
dark wash straight-leg jeans
black mules   ⟶ for work and play
basic light-gray sweater

MEDIUM PRIORITY

white jumpsuit
chambray shirt
daytime bag (crossbody)
charcoal blazer for work
two more tops for work
midlength skirt
     ⟶ (must be a thick fabric like wool or tweed)

LOW PRIORITY

black beret
one or two comfy pants for lounging at home
another clutch bag (fun statement piece!)
new tennis shorts
black platform boots
red cardigan or lightweight jacket

STEP 4: OVERHAUL YOUR WARDROBE ONE ITEM AT A TIME

Think of your list of priorities as your personal shopping compass. Start from the top and find a great version of your highest-priority item. Then, work your way further down your list, however fast or slow your budget allows.

And remember: Your shopping list isn't set in stone. Feel free to add more items or details about existing items, delete others, or reorganize your priorities as you discover more about your style.

Top three overhaul mistakes to avoid

MISTAKE 1: COMPROMISING ON QUALITY FOR A LOWER PRICE

If your wardrobe still needs a lot of work, you may at some point feel tempted to go ahead and buy a bunch of so-so but affordable pieces just to have *more* to wear. Don't do it! Remember that your goal is to end up with a high-quality wardrobe that you can wear and love for many seasons to come. By compromising on crucial things like a great fit or a comfortable material, and knowingly buying something that won't last long or that you'll eventually want to replace, you are jumping straight back into the same vicious cycle you are trying to break out of.

> If you are on a tight budget, that's all the more reason to use your money well and not spread it across lots of imperfect things.

Make it your mission to always find a great-quality version for each item on your list. Now, that does *not* mean that everything you buy needs to be expensive (read more about the shaky relationship between garment quality and price on pages 224–225). But for some big-ticket items like a great leather jacket or a winter coat, it may mean you can buy only one item this month or even this season. And that's okay because over time you'll end up with a great selection of high-quality pieces that you can wear for many years to come.

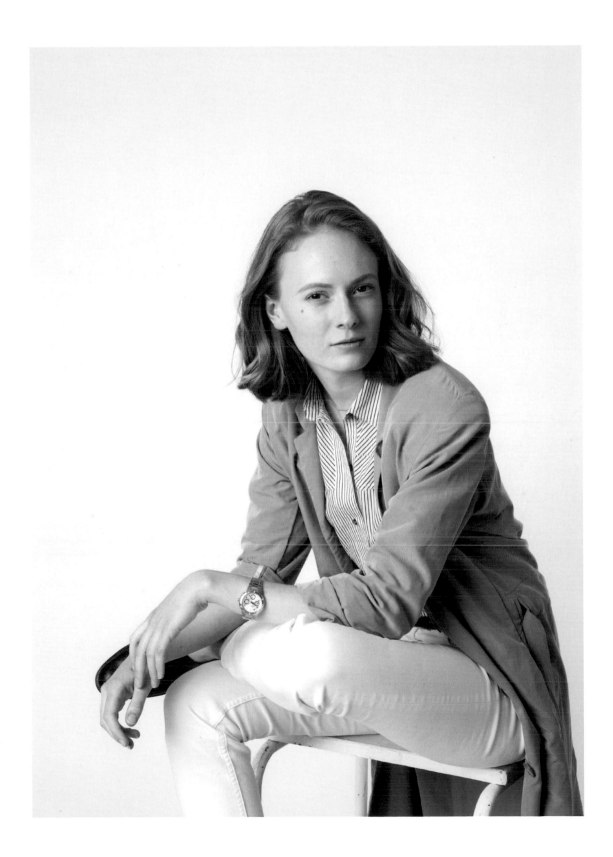

MISTAKE 2: BUYING YOURSELF AN ENTIRELY NEW WARDROBE ALL AT ONCE

If you want to completely revamp your wardrobe (and, say, go from your standard jeans-and-tee combo to a more edgy, glamorous chic), it may also seem like a good idea to just buy yourself a whole new wardrobe all at once, Cinderella-style.

The danger here is of course that, as with any extreme makeover, you'll rush it, not think things through properly, and subsequently end up with a whole closet full of stuff that you *thought* you would like, but that in the end just doesn't quite feel like *you*.

Because even if you spent a good chunk of time defining your new style and were extra diligent during the experimentation stage, you can never predict with 100 percent accuracy how you'll feel wearing a completely different look in real life. And that's why the more you want to change your wardrobe's overall aesthetic, the slower you should go. Because each new piece gives you a chance to recalibrate the overall style direction in which you are heading.

And as you revamp your wardrobe, slowly and piece by piece, you are also giving yourself ample time to adjust to your new look emotionally and grow into it. Because the second major risk of shotgun makeovers is that you may not feel quite like yourself, as if you're wearing a costume.

The moral of the story is there's nothing wrong with aiming for a total wardrobe revamp, but do it gradually. Buy one piece in your new style and wear it with the rest of your wardrobe for a while and see how you feel. Then add another new piece and so on.

MISTAKE 3: BUYING A TON OF NEW CLOTHES JUST BEFORE A MAJOR LIFESTYLE CHANGE

This one is closely related to mistake 2 but deserves a special mention because it's all too common!

Starting a new job, having a baby, or moving to a new city—if there's a big change coming up in your life, it's only natural that you want to be well prepared and stock your wardrobe in advance with a few new pieces. And that's totally fine. What's not such a good idea is spending a lot of money on new clothes just before a major lifestyle change, especially if you want to use that change as an opportunity to revamp your look.

Before I moved to London for grad school I bought at least five pairs of high heels. During college I probably wore heels a total of three times, but I thought, "London is a fashion capital—now is my chance to up my fashion game!" And guess what happened: I ended up selling every single pair on eBay because I'm a flats girl at heart, even in fashion-forward London.

We all have preconceived ideas about what it's like to live a certain lifestyle. But unless you yourself have been in that situation, it's impossible to predict exactly how you'll feel, what the atmosphere and the people around you will be like, and, consequently, what you will want to wear.

If you've already had a baby and know you lived in maxi dresses and cardigans during your last pregnancy, go ahead and fill up your wardrobe with those pieces again now that baby number two is on its way. But if you are moving to New York City and you have never lived in a big city before, it's better to wait before spending a lot of money. Wait a few weeks and suss out what your new life is really like. Then repeat the lifestyle analysis from page 106 and use the results as the basis for your wardrobe overhaul.

HOW TO DEAL WHEN SHOPPING OVERWHELMS

"I love fashion but I hate buying clothes." What sounds like a paradox is actually a pretty common sentiment.

The combination of way too many options and a public setting (read: more pressure) make stores a powerhouse of overwhelming experiences and choice anxiety. If you have a tendency to feel stressed, awkward, or anxious while shopping and it's keeping you from making the best choices you can—or even from buying any new clothes at all—this section is for you. If you're a die-hard shopaholic and can't think of a more fun way to spend your Saturday afternoon than to shop, then feel free to skip this page.

THE BASICS

- Don't shop during rush hour. A big factor that makes shopping a stressful experience for many is being surrounded by people, which adds a certain amount of social pressure and raises stress hormone levels. And more people equals more stress, so avoid going shopping during notoriously busy time slots (that includes early evenings, lunchtime, and weekend afternoons). Weekday mid-mornings are usually the quietest. If you work nine to five, try going early on a weekend.
- Don't shop when you are tired, sad, or otherwise not feeling well. Wear a favorite outfit for an extra boost of confidence.
- Wear something that's comfortable and easy to take off and put back on.

SHOP ONLINE!

The easiest way to circumvent all the stress of shopping is to simply do it online. That way you can take all time in the world to browse and compare your options and can even see how the pieces you have ordered look with the rest of your wardrobe. Plus, your lighting at home is always going to be nicer and more flattering than the bright fluorescent light in your standard fitting room.

But of course, shopping online isn't always the more practical option and, in some cases, going to an actual store may actually be quicker, and less of a hassle when you want to try on a ton of clothes from multiple brands, have no idea what size to order, or don't want to deal with returns. Here are three easy techniques to help you banish overwhelming shopping experiences for those situations.

ANTISTRESS TIPS FOR SHOPPING IN PERSON

Tip 1: Set mini goals

When we feel overwhelmed, it's usually because (1) the task at hand seems too hard or (2) the task is unclear. That's why, as a "nervous shopper," your best bet is to make the whole experience as easy and fail-proof as possible. Don't force yourself to go on three-hour shopping trips. Instead, choose one or two stores that you want to visit and predetermine what type of clothes you'll look at too.

For example, try on button-down shirts and look at sunglasses in shops A and B. Or, find five sweaters in different colors to try on in store X. Make it super specific and super doable. Ignore everything else. Then set another mini goal and repeat.

Tip 2: Research possible buys before you hit the shops

Have you ever heard of the *paradox of choice*? It's a term coined by psychologist Barry Schwartz and describes how we as consumers typically end up feeling *less* satisfied and more anxious about our choice when we have *more* options.

Most stores nowadays have a huge selection of clothes on display, making them a major source of shopper's anxiety. If you are already prone to feeling anxious in stores, you need to find a way to artificially limit your options.

The easiest way to do this is to simply spend a bit of time online beforehand. Browse the online shops of brands and stores you're considering and pick a small number of pieces to try on. That way you can just head straight for your mini preselection at the store and ignore everything else.

Tip 3: Postpone your decision until you are back home

To buy or not to buy: When it comes to making a decision, some people get so overwhelmed and stressed out that they drop everything and leave or, even worse, buy whatever they have in their hands right then, just to be able to get out of that store. If that sounds like you, try this little technique the next time you need new clothes:

Enter a store, but decide beforehand that you are not going to buy *anything*. Your goal for this visit is solely to collect information. Try on a handful of pieces, inspect from all angles, and take pictures with your phone while you're in the dressing room. Then, just leave. Once you are back home you can go back over all the information you have collected at your own pace and make your decision without feeling pressured.

14/

How (and when) to build a capsule wardrobe

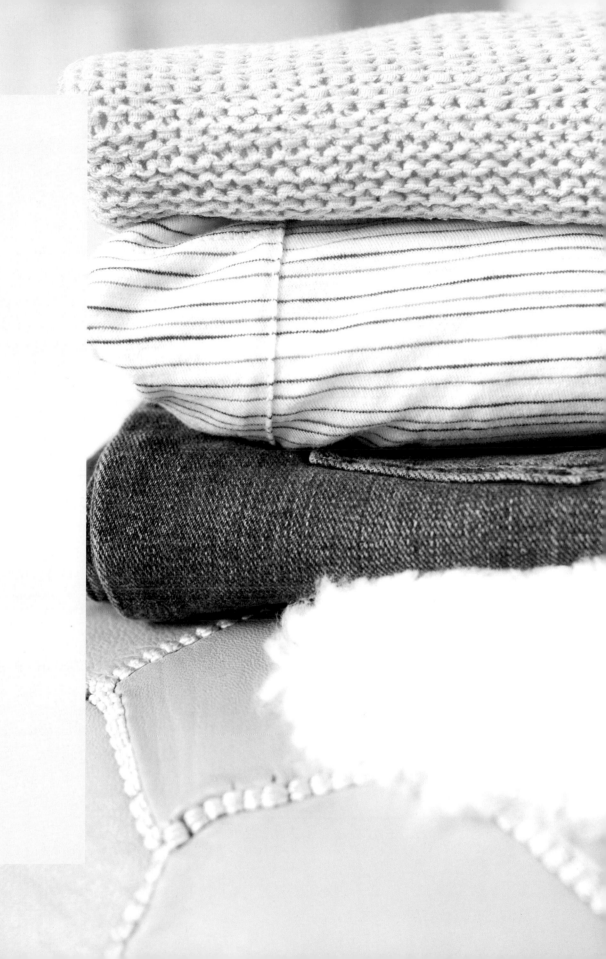

If you love the idea of owning a small collection of perfectly interchangeable clothes, this chapter is for you! Learn all about capsule wardrobes, including how to curate your own in six simple steps.

So far, our focus in this part of this book has been on your entire closet: how to detox it, how to improve it, and how to overhaul it piece by piece. But you can use the same tools and techniques you've learned in previous chapters to perfect just a small subsection of your closet: a capsule wardrobe.

What is a capsule wardrobe?

The concept of the capsule wardrobe has become more and more popular in recent years, but actually, it's been around for a while.

THE ORIGINAL CAPSULE WARDROBE

Originally, the term *capsule wardrobe* was coined sometime in the 1970s by British style guru Suzie Faux. Up until then, most women had whole outfits hanging in their closets rather than interchangeable pieces. Having a capsule wardrobe—several timeless items that never go out of style and that can be combined with seasonal fashion—was considered new and exciting at the time, perfect for the modern working woman. Commonly recommended pieces for capsule wardrobes were things like pencil skirts, white button-downs, and other plain and therefore versatile separates. Essentially, capsule wardrobe pieces used to have the function of what I call *basics* in this book.

THE CAPSULE WARDROBE NOW

Nowadays, what we think of as a capsule wardrobe is a little different. Here's a quick overview:

- A capsule wardrobe consists of twenty to forty pieces including shoes and outerwear (but that number doesn't include accessories or specialty items like underwear, gym gear, or sleepwear).
- It is is intended to be a stand-alone wardrobe, that is, you generally don't mix your capsule wardrobe pieces with the rest of your clothes.
- Since you wear only a small selection of pieces, you need to regularly rebuild your capsule wardrobe to keep it tailored to the current weather season. Each time you rebuild your capsule wardrobe, you pick clothes from your entire closet (or from storage). Once you've made your choices, all your other clothes are on hiatus until it's time for the next season. Your capsule wardrobe is essentially the "active" part of your entire closet.

"How Big Should My Capsule Wardrobe Be?"

The ideal size of your capsule wardrobe depends on three factors—style, lifestyle, and need for variety:

- **Style:** If you like simple outfits, you will need *fewer pieces* than someone who loves a layered look.
- **Lifestyle:** If you have to dress for a range of different occasions, you will need *more pieces* than someone who can wear the same type of outfits every day.
- **Need for variety:** If you like having lots of options, you will need *more pieces* than someone who doesn't mind repeating outfits relatively frequently.

Bottom line: There is no one perfect number. Feel free to aim for a range as you set out to build your capsule wardrobe, whether it's twenty to twenty-five or "around forty" pieces, but be prepared to adjust that number if necessary.

Why build a capsule wardrobe?

A commonly touted benefit of capsule wardrobes is that they make it easier to choose outfits in the morning because all the pieces in your wardrobe work well with each other. Building a capsule wardrobe is also supposed to be a great way to become a smarter, more thoughtful shopper. And all of that is true! But here's the thing: if you work with the techniques in this book, you'll get the same result. You don't need to limit yourself to a low number of pieces to dress well, have a closet of pieces that all work well together, or curb impulse shopping. You can achieve those things no matter how many clothes you want to keep in your closet. In fact, for some people, forty pieces is close or even above the number they would wear either way (keep in mind we're excluding things like underwear, accessories, and special occasion clothes here). In that case, their wardrobe is both a capsule and a regular wardrobe, and it doesn't really matter what they choose to call it.

So why build a capsule wardrobe at all? Why consciously choose to limit what you are wearing? From my experience, there are five types of people who do well with the concept. If you are one of them, consider giving it a try!

YOU LOVE SIMPLICITY

Some people (myself included) simply like the idea of owning a perfectly curated small set of clothes. In her book *Better Than Before* author Gretchen Rubin calls this group of people *simplicity lovers*. They derive a sense of pleasure from organizing and getting rid of things and are easily overwhelmed by too much going on around them. On the other end of the spectrum there are the *abundance lovers*, who like having lots of options and variety. They are often avid collectors and their living space is usually overflowing with stuff and decorative tidbits. If you are an abundance lover, the thought of limiting your wardrobe to a small set of clothes will sound stifling to you. But if you are a simplicity lover, it's right up your alley!

YOUR WARDROBE STILL NEEDS A LOT OF WORK

If your current wardrobe contains barely any clothes you like, it can be helpful to aim for a capsule wardrobe first rather than a complete closet overhaul. It's the difference between organizing a small get-together with friends and planning a multiday wedding weekend with five hundred guests. There are less moving parts to worry about and you'll reach your goal sooner. You'll end up with a stand-alone, functional core set of clothes that you can then expand on or just keep wearing as is.

YOU WANT TO GET MORE CREATIVE AND MAKE THE MOST OF YOUR EXISTING CLOTHES

If you find yourself shopping for new stuff whenever you're out of outfit ideas, building a capsule wardrobe is a great way to challenge yourself to make more out of the clothes you already have. Have you heard of the "30x30 Remix"? It's a fun wardrobe challenge made popular by Kendi Skeen of the blog *Kendi Everyday*. Here's how it works: you choose thirty pieces from your entire closet and then try to build thirty different outfits with your thirty pieces throughout the next month. Of course you can also just choose twenty pieces and do it for twenty days, or wear thirty pieces in as many different ways as you can for three whole months. It's up to you!

YOU HAVE TO STICK TO A DRESS CODE FOR WORK

As mentioned on page 152, I recommend building a separate wardrobe for work if you have to adhere to a dress code or just want to wear a different style during business hours. That way you're free to fully express your own personal style during your free time *and* have a set of perfectly functional and appropriate clothes for work.

YOU ARE TRAVELING OR HAVE A BUSY FEW MONTHS AHEAD

Having a lot of options isn't always a good thing, especially when you're ridiculously busy and don't want to waste what little time you do have in front of your closet deciding what to wear, or if you are living out of a suitcase. Whenever I have a busy month of traveling or work coming up, I put together a versatile twenty-piece capsule wardrobe that will work for all the different activities I have planned. I've done this many times over the last few years, and it's always been a huge time- and energy-saver because I can literally just grab an outfit and go in the morning. You can use the same trick to save time as you finish up your thesis, spend time at home with your newborn, hustle through the busiest time of year for your business, or travel for an extended period of time. Do a little bit of extra planning up front to build a flexible, versatile wardrobe and then feel free to forget all about your clothes for a while, because it's already been taken care of.

"How Often Should I Rebuild My Capsule Wardrobe?"

The answer depends on why you built your capsule wardrobe in the first place. If you want to keep wearing a capsule wardrobe for the foreseeable future, either because you love the simplicity of it or have a work capsule, a good time frame to rebuild is every three months, to keep your wardrobe tailored to the weather. When I was still regularly wearing a capsule wardrobe, I would rebuild it at the beginning of every October, January, April, and July—just before each new season. Skip to chapter 21 to read more about how to maintain and update your closet year-round.

If your goal is to get more creative when it comes to using the clothes you already have, you may choose to rebuild your capsule wardrobe more frequently, for example every one or two months. That way you can include different pieces each time and eventually get to know your entire closet.

And of course, if you just want to wear a capsule wardrobe for a fixed period of time, for example while you travel or finish up a big project, you don't have to rebuild your capsule at all and can simply go back to wearing your entire closet as normal.

And remember: Rebuilding your capsule wardrobe does not mean *buying* a whole new wardrobe. Instead, take your pick from everything you have in your closet and in storage right now, and then, if you are still missing a few crucial pieces to round everything out, go ahead and buy them.

How to build a capsule wardrobe

Essentially, a capsule wardrobe is just a regular wardrobe in a mini format, and you can use all the same techniques we've talked about so far to build it.

The only extra tip I have for you is this: the more carefully you plan your capsule and select your pieces, the better.

If you want to keep your capsule wardrobe below a certain size and be functional at the same time, every piece really needs to pull its weight. There is no leeway, no room for pieces that you only kinda like or that work only as part of a single outfit, like sparkly statement tops that you might get to wear once a month. Each piece in your capsule should fit your style 100 percent, be practical, and be something that you can wear in lots of different ways, multiple times in a month or even in a week.

Here is the general process I recommend you use to create your capsule wardrobe, along with the relevant chapters in this book:

STEP 1: DEFINE THE ACTIVITIES FOR WHICH YOUR WARDROBE SHOULD BE TAILORED

If you have already created a pie chart for your everyday lifestyle (as shown on page 108), you can simply use that as the basis for your capsule wardrobe. Create a separate pie chart if you are building a capsule solely for work or a specific time period where you'll be wearing different clothes than you usually do (such as for traveling).

> Relevant chapter: Chapter 8, How to build a wardrobe that fits your real life (not your fantasy life) (page 102)

STEP 2: CREATE A MINI STYLE PROFILE

Your capsule wardrobe style profile should be a more defined version of the style profile you have already created for your overall personal style on page 85. Make it as specific as possible ("light blue and pistachio" instead of "cool pastel shades") and tailor it to your pie chart of activities and the weather. Also keep in mind that your style profile will need to be smaller in range: you have only a limited number of pieces to implement it with, so instead of including six different fabrics for example, choose two or three favorites that work well with each other, so you can mix and match all your pieces.

> Relevant chapter: Chapter 6, Putting it all together: your style profile (page 78)

STEP 3: CREATE A BASIC WARDROBE STRUCTURE

Based on your pie chart and your mini stye profile, write down a structure for your capsule wardrobe that specifies how many pieces it should include of every item category: for example, jeans, tops, sneakers, and so on. Definitely include your outfit formula ingredients as item categories and any other types of items you like to wear regularly. Use the laundry ratio technique from page 145 to figure out an optimal number of pieces for each item category, based on how often they need to be washed.

Here's an example of what your basic wardrobe structure could look like:

- Straight-cut jeans: 2
- Wide-leg pants: 2
- Skirts: 2
- Coats: 1
- Jackets: 1

- Blazers: 2
- Cardigans: 4
- Knit sweaters: 5
- Tank tops: 4
- Long-sleeve T-shirts: 3

- Loafers: 1
- Pumps: 2
- Sneakers: 1

Relevant chapter: Chapter 11, Working with outfit formulas (page 138)

STEP 4: ADD DETAIL TO YOUR STRUCTURE

Next, go through your closet to pick out any items you definitely want to include in your capsule wardrobe and add these to your structure (as long as they work with the mini profile and the pie chart of activities you created).

Then, figure out what you want each missing piece to look like, in terms of its color, material, silhouette, and so on. To make sure your missing pieces form a versatile, mixable capsule wardrobe in combination with the pieces you already own, it can be helpful to refer to any of the three strategies I showed you in chapters 9 to 11: closet composition, color palettes, and outfit formulas.

Be prepared to go back and forth a couple of times between picking out clothes from your closet and defining missing items, until you have found a good mix.

Here is what your capsule wardrobe structure might look like after this step:

2 PAIRS OF STRAIGHT-CUT JEANS
- Dark-wash √
- Medium wash √

2 PAIRS OF WIDE-LEG PANTS
- Black √
- White √

2 SKIRTS
- Forest-green pencil √
- Gray mini with lace hemline

1 COAT
- Gray wool √

1 JACKET
- Medium-wash denim √

2 BLAZERS
- Black √
- White

4 CARDIGANS
- Forest-green √
- Plum (long-line) √
- Black √
- Dusty rose

5 KNIT SWEATERS
- White cable knit √
- White with lace appliqué
- Gray √
- Embellished black sweater √
- Plum/rose Fair Isle

4 TANK TOPS
- Black satin √
- Gray cotton √
- White
- Black/white sequinned √

3 LONG-SLEEVE T-SHIRTS
- White/navy striped √
- Gray dolman √
- Simple black V neck √

1 PAIR OF LOAFERS
- Black with tassels √

2 PAIRS OF PUMPS
- Black K
- Plum √

1 PAIR OF SNEAKERS
- Gray √

√ = What I own already

Relevant chapters: Chapter 9, Closet composition 101 (page 112); Chapter 10, Selecting a versatile color palette (page 124); Chapter 11, Working with outfit formulas (page 138); Chapter 12, Business hours: tweaking your wardrobe for work (page 148)

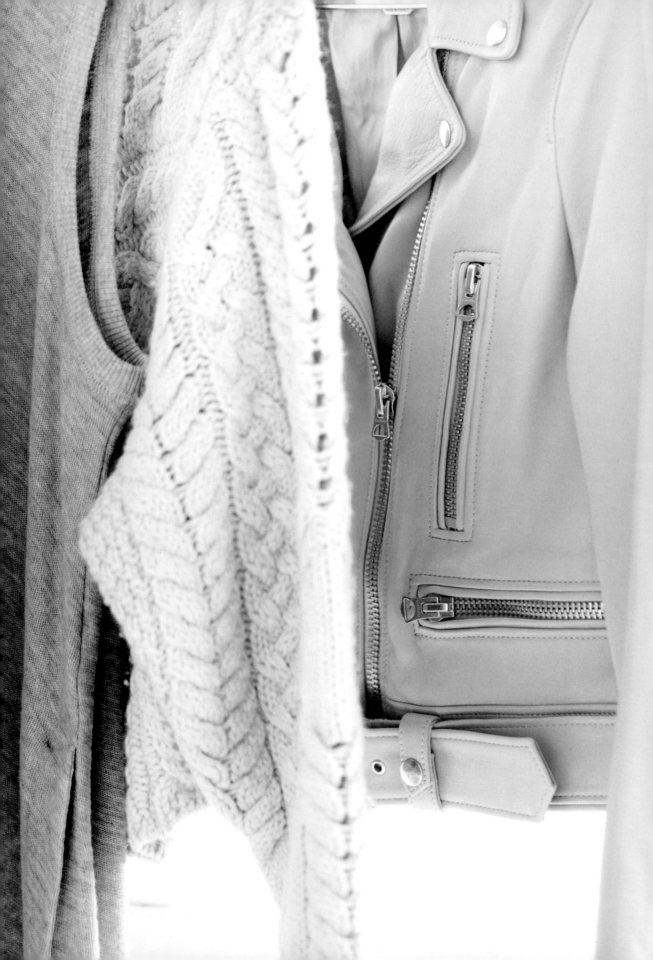

STEP 5: WRITE A SHOPPING LIST

Now that you know what you want your capsule wardrobe to look like, you can follow the four-step overhaul I described in chapter 13 to implement it and prioritize missing pieces.

> Relevant chapter: Chapter 13, Overhauling your wardrobe: a step-by-step road map (page 158)

STEP 6: PLAN OUTFITS

Reserve some time to get to know your new capsule wardrobe inside out and come up with a repertoire of go-to looks.

> Relevant chapter: Chapter 15, Become your own best stylist (page 182)

15/
Become your own best stylist

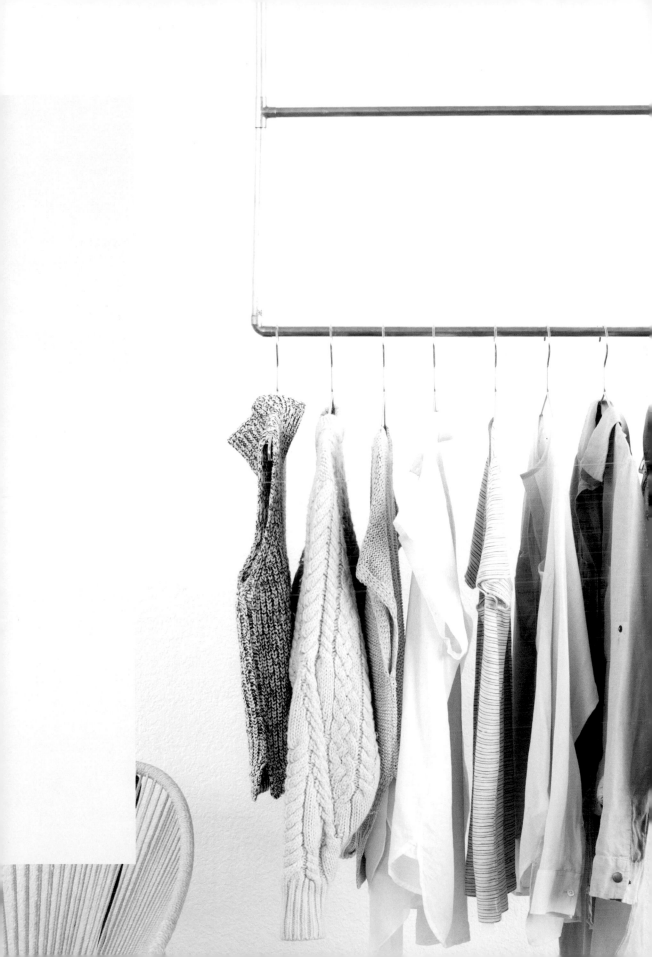

Get to know your new-and-improved wardrobe inside out, build up an arsenal of styling tricks, and challenge yourself to come up with a bunch of new go-to looks that all reflect your personal style perfectly.

Building a great outfit is like cooking a yummy dish: you need high-quality ingredients but then you also need to combine them the right way and add the right spices.

If you've just overhauled your wardrobe or added a few new pieces, you've already stocked your pantry with lots of great ingredients. Now, as the last step on the road to your perfect wardrobe, it's time to figure out how to best use those ingredients to build outfits that are 100 percent in tune with your personal style.

You should conduct a fitting after a major wardrobe overhaul, biannually as part of your preseason wardrobe prep and whenever you want to switch up your look.

So get ready to flex your styling muscles and reserve at least two hours for a fitting! A fitting? Yep!

Costume designers and fashion stylists host fittings with their clients to test-drive all the outfits needed for an event or on set, and they tweak, tailor, and fine-tune them to perfection. Even if you don't have a big awards show to go to any time soon, you can still use that same hands-on approach to familiarize yourself with your new wardrobe, learn how to make the most of it, and become your own best stylist.

What to do during your fitting

Your mission is to get creative, experiment, and play dress-up! Try on a ton of combinations and fine-tune them using accessories and other styling tricks until you've come up with a bunch of new looks that you can't wait to wear.

WHAT YOU NEED

- The mood board you created to summarize your personal style (for reference)
- A full-length mirror
- A camera or your smartphone
- Your style file for note taking
- A favorite upbeat playlist of music

Start each new outfit by first picking your main ingredients: pants, tops, shoes, and so on. Use your outfit formulas as a guideline, or just put together a good mix of basics, key pieces, and statement pieces. Once you are happy with your ensemble, garnish it! Add a dainty necklace, belt, cute scarf, or stack of bangles. Scrunch up your sleeves, put on a bright red lipstick or a cat eye (or both), and tie a shirt around your waist. (Check out page 189 for a list of styling tricks.)

BUILD A REPERTOIRE OF FAVORITE LOOKS

Fine-tune your outfits until they are 100 percent *your* style. Then snap a picture of your look and take notes. Throughout your fitting, pay attention to two things:

1. The main ingredients: Which pieces go well with each other?
2. The spices: What styling tricks (including accessories) work best with each of your items?

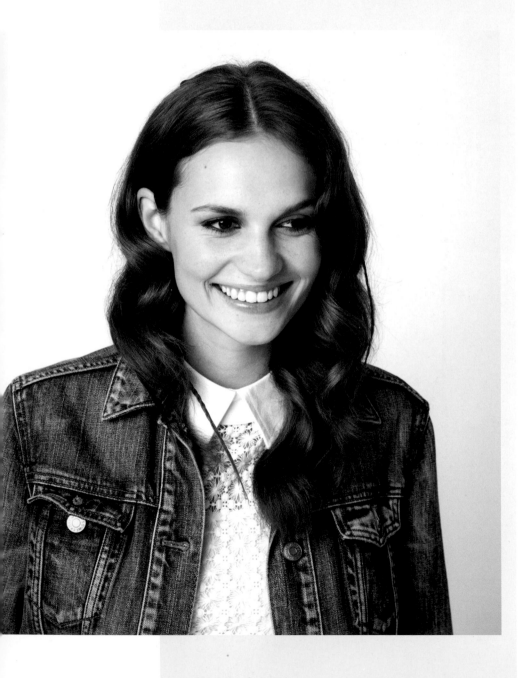

Styling challenges

Complete these challenges as part of your fitting or whenever you need some fresh new ideas. Start by tackling the three foundation-level challenges. They will help you get to know the basic structure of your wardrobe. After that, pick a few of the advanced-level challenges to dig even deeper.

FOUNDATION LEVEL

- **Inaugurate new pieces.** No matter whether you've just finished a major wardrobe overhaul or just bought a couple of fresh pieces for the new season, make sure you spend a little bit of time getting to know each new item and find out as much as possible about it: what occasions could you wear it to, with what other pieces does it go well, and what type of styling brings out the best in it? Find at least three different ways to wear each new piece and make sure you record all your findings in your style file.

- **Get to know your outfit formulas.** Pick one of your outfit formulas and use it to put together five different looks. Use accessories, additional pieces, and styling tricks to add variety and differentiate between them.

- **Put your key pieces to work.** Choose your five most important key pieces and challenge yourself to create three outfits, each as different from each other as possible. For example, your perfect black blazer might already work really well for daytime, but let's see if you can also make it work as part of a super-casual weekend look or a fancier going-out-at-night outfit.

ADVANCED LEVEL

- **Style a plain base look five different ways.** Start with an outfit of basics, like black jeans and a simple white top. Then challenge yourself to transform that base layer into five completely different looks, using accessories, additional pieces, hair and makeup, and other styling tricks.

- **Create a flagship look.** Condense your entire personal style into a single outfit. Fine-tune every detail, including jewelry and makeup.

- **Style three weekend looks.** What are your favorite things to do on the weekends? Build three outfits that are perfect for those activities.

- **Style three work looks.** Time for business. Put together a few different outfits that you could wear the next time you have an important meeting or a big presentation and want to feel ultra confident.

- **Dress it up, dress it down.** Start out with one of your go-to looks and then dress it either up or down by amping up or toning down its individual elements one by one, by adding, removing, or changing your makeup; adding or removing accessories; tucking in hemlines; switching out your shoes; adding a different jacket; and so on. See how far you can take it in either direction.

- **Play a game of six degrees of separation.** To get started, pick two complete outfits (no overlapping pieces). Next, start out with one of your looks and see if you can create another equally great look by switching out a single item, two at the most. Continue to create new outfits by switching out one or two pieces each time, until you have eventually linked your two starting outfits.
- **Style a week's worth of outfits with only ten pieces.** This is a two-part challenge, because you need to flex your styling muscles to style your pieces in different ways, and you also need to choose the right pieces in the first place. But once you have found a versatile set of pieces, packing for your next trip will be super easy.

Build an arsenal of styling tricks

Look closely at any great outfit you see in magazines or on blogs and you'll notice the huge amount of detail and thought that went into it. That gorgeous dress an actress is wearing is made all the more beautiful by her red lipstick and sapphire green earrings. That cozy but ultra chic fall outfit in the September issue of your favorite magazine wouldn't look half as good without the belt, the layering, the tote bag, and the boots with socks peeking out from them. And even if the outfit consists of nothing but a T-shirt and a pair of jeans, or is otherwise simple and minimalist, little details like the cuffing of the jeans, the tuck of the T-shirt, or the rolling of the sleeves can take it to the next level.

Styling is what turns a good outfit into a great one.

While the process of styling an outfit may seem elusive, it's actually quite simple because there are only so many basic elements that can be *adjusted* or *added to* an outfit (see the list on the next page).

Some of these will work for your unique personal style and help you take your outfits to the next level; others won't. As you experiment with different outfit combinations during your fitting, make it a point to also throw as many different styling tricks into the mix as you can to see which ones you like the best.

Start by testing out the styling techniques you discovered during your inspiration search and fieldwork stage, but then branch out. Take notes about what type of pieces go particularly well with what type of styling techniques. Also, try to pay attention to what effect a certain styling trick has so you can use it to calibrate any look.

 Write a list of your favorite styling tricks and add to it whenever you come across a new idea you might want to try.

- **Tucking in shirts:** Adds structure and interest to your outfit. Experiment with full tucks, front tucks, and half tucks.
- **Cuffing pants:** This can mean anything from skinny half-rolled cuffs to a solid 2-inch cuff.
- **Rolling up sleeves:** This works for jackets and shirts, as well as for long- and short-sleeve tops alike.
- **Belts:** From skinny to wide, worn up high on the natural waistline, low on the hips, or anything in between.
- **Scarves:** From silk handkerchiefs to blanket scarves.
- **Jewelry:** Necklaces, bracelets or bangles, rings, earrings, and brooches.
- **Other accessories:** Glasses or sunglasses, tights, hair accessories, hats, and gloves.
- **Layers:** Think adding an accent top that peeks out around the neckline, hemline, or sleeve openings. Or, try tying a shirt around your waist or hips.
- **Makeup and hair styling:** These are important parts of your look, whether you prefer a bold or neutral lip color, an updo or a looser hair look.

PART IV

THE ART OF SHOPPING

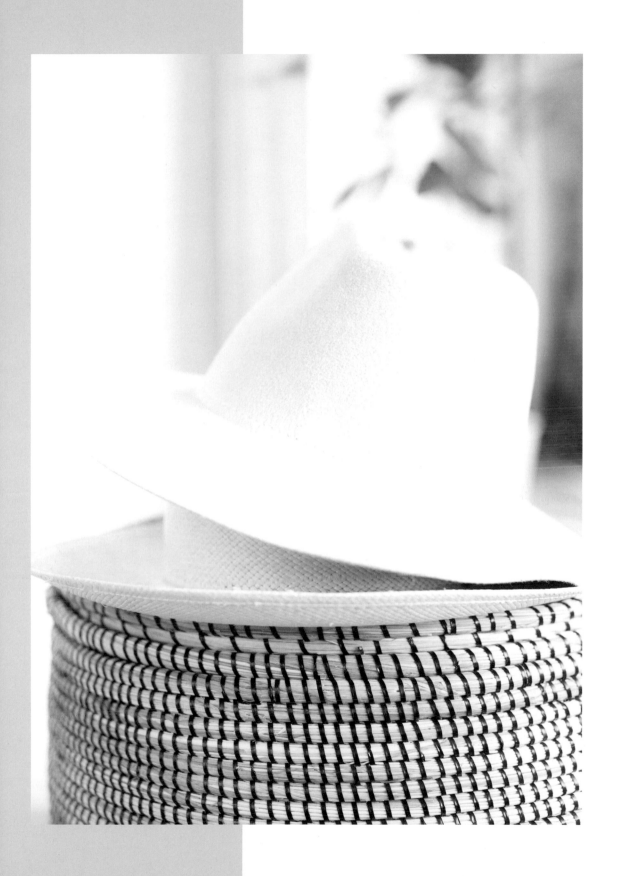

16/

How to shop like a conscious consumer

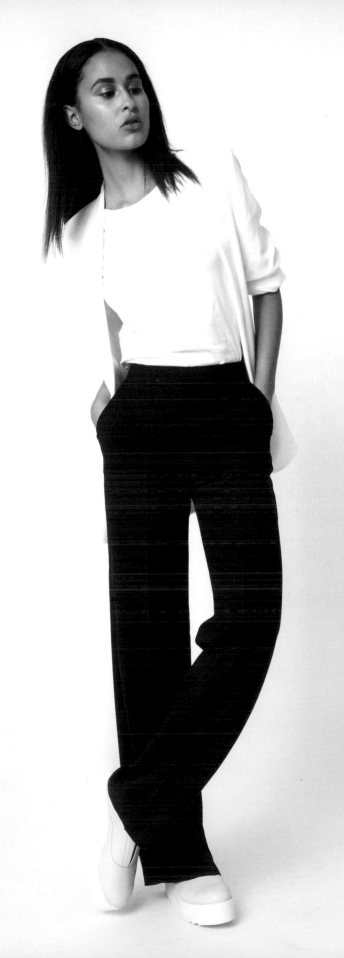

The definitive guide to smart shopping: Escape the fast fashion cycle, find pieces you love, and prevent impulse buys with these three essential habits.

Being a conscious consumer in a world that's obsessed with amassing more and more stuff can be a real challenge. Glossy billboards, highly produced celebrity-driven ads, and clever social media campaigns are everywhere, and stylish clothing is now more accessible and affordable than ever. This is a dangerous combination that has had quite the impact on our spending habits: The average person in the 1960s bought fewer than twenty-five new garments a year and spent almost 10 percent of his or her income on clothes. Nowadays, we buy close to seventy new pieces a year—more than one per week—but spend less than 3.5 percent of our income on clothes.

We buy more but invest less per piece. And I'm not just talking about money. We also invest less time and thought into each purchase. Why? Because we can. With the rise of the fast-fashion industry, the average prices for wearables have dropped steadily and we simply no longer have to think twice about every piece we buy. But lower prices aren't the only reason for our haphazard spending.

The new normal

In recent years, there has been a huge shift in the way we use technology. We are online and "connected" 24/7, and that has made it a lot easier for brands to reach us. Instead of having to rely on expensive magazine ads or the persuasive powers of their sales assistants, brands can now simply send out a few tweets and sponsor a few bloggers to reach a global audience of millions.

As a result, the online world is so saturated with ads and brand messages, it's impossible to escape. And so most of us spend our days surrounded by pretty pictures of stuff and glamorous people talking about that stuff. Every day, we see fashion bloggers and Instagrammers buying more and more, without thinking about it too much. And even if at first we think, "What, you bought *another* pair of leopard heels?!" over time that constant exposure changes our own perception of what's normal and we ourselves get used to buying more and more without thinking about it too much. Flash sales, two-for-one deals, and constantly changing collections teach us to make fast decisions. Being less selective becomes the new normal.

Escaping the cycle

The way you shop is nothing but a set of habits you have picked up over the years. And if you want to change the way you shop and become more selective and thoughtful about what you buy and what goes into your wardrobe, then you need to gradually replace those habits with some new ones.

Most women I know who have successfully escaped the fast-fashion cycle and now own personalized, well-curated wardrobes all follow the same general process when it comes to shopping for new pieces. That process can be broken down into three key habits, which I'll walk you through in this chapter.

None of these habits require drastic measures or huge amounts of willpower, so don't worry—you don't have to unfollow half of your Instagram list, vow to never shop at your favorite budget store again, or go on a thirty-day shopping fast to become a more selective, thoughtful shopper. Instead, it's all about slowing down the process and subtly tweaking the way you shop, to give you both more energy and deliberation time to make better purchasing decisions.

HABIT 1: WRITE DETAILED SHOPPING LISTS

Have you ever noticed how most fashion stores are set up in the same way? Fashion-forward, higher-priced pieces are in the front and on mannequins so you definitely won't miss them, the permanent collection is in the back, and the way to the register is always conveniently lined with budget-friendly goodies for you to grab while you wait. No matter whether you shop at Forever 21 or Anthropologie, that's the setup you will find 95 percent of the time because it's what brings in the most sales. After decades of research and number crunching, brands know exactly how to lure us in, point us toward the pricy stuff, and send us home with way more than we came in for.

Your best defense is a clear, succinct shopping list (like the one you created in your style file in preparation for your wardrobe overhaul). Get in the habit of deciding what you want to buy *before* you hit the shops, online or in person at a brick-and-mortar store.

The average shopper does the exact opposite: they go on a little shopping trip as soon as they have a vague idea of what they want to buy ("pants," "fancy outfit," "something blue") and then let external circumstances fill in the details. What they eventually take home is above all a result of chance, which items caught their attention, what was on sale, what the nice sales assistant talked them into, and how many stores they made it to until their feet started to hurt.

And sure, sometimes serendipity strikes and that approach works out just fine. But when you're trying to build a cohesive wardrobe, your shopping process really needs to be more strategic than that, because you're not just looking for any old pair of pants—you need one with specific qualities that work with the rest of your clothes, your color palette, and your style profile and that matches your preferences for things like fabric composition, fit, and silhouette.

And the more you can define these qualities in advance, the better off you will be when you do eventually go out to shop. You'll be able to do a quick online search for items that fit your criteria and put together a short list of brands. You'll be able to narrow down your list of go-to shops. And then, once you are in a store, you'll be able to use your predefined criteria like a filter to scan what's available.

All this not only increases the likelihood that you'll actually find what you are looking for, but it also helps to de-stress the entire process and preserve your energy, thereby keeping you from settling for something you're not all that crazy about.

And of course, having a good idea about what exactly it is you are looking for is also the best way to avoid impulse buys because it gives you a clear focus, a target. While you are concentrating on hunting down that target, you are much less likely to get sidetracked by any of the other pretty things on display that may look cute but wouldn't work with your wardrobe right now, let alone fit into your budget.

So the next time you are considering adding something new to your wardrobe, take a couple of minutes to figure out exactly what kind of garment you are looking for, using your style profile, color palette, outfit formulas, and any other basic parameters you have set for your wardrobe.

Key factors to consider when writing a shopping list:

- Overall style
- Color
- Cut, silhouette, and fit
- Material

- Details
- Sleeve length
- Neckline
- Pattern

Feel free to add as much info as you want to your shopping list, but make sure you distinguish between qualities that are a must (such as white or eggshell color, cotton fabric) and those that aren't essential but nice to have (such as a crew neckline).

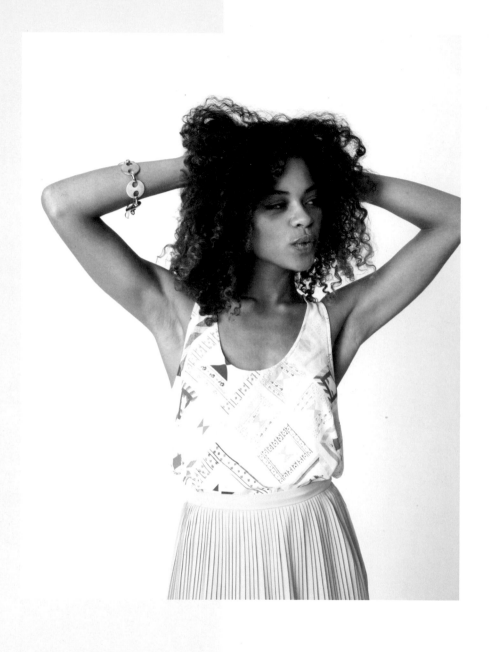

HABIT 2: TAKE IT SLOW

Compared to the average shopper, people who own carefully curated wardrobes shop at a snail's pace. They like to take their time to compare all options before they make a decision and will rarely buy a piece on the same day they first spotted it in a store or online.

Again, it all boils down to being selective. If you are looking for a very specific piece, one that ticks all your checkboxes in terms of style, fit, details, and so on, one shopping trip will usually not give you enough time to consider a possible new garment from all angles.

> By deliberately taking it slow, you are giving yourself the chance to be thorough and make sure you aren't rushing your decision or acting on impulse.

So instead of checking off all your shopping on a single afternoon, try this approach: take your time to define exactly what type of item you need and write a very specific shopping list. Then check out some of your favorite brands online and see if any of them offer a piece that fits your criteria. Put together a short list of items that you can try on in a nearby store or just order directly (making sure that you can return any items that don't work out). Read reviews and search for pictures of the piece online. How does it look as part of an outfit? What are people saying about the fabric?

Once you have tried on the items on your short list, compare each piece to your list of criteria and think about how well they each would work as part of your current wardrobe. Take a walk around the block if you are not sure or put the items on hold and sleep on it. If none of your final contenders feel quite right, just walk away. It's better to live with a gap in your wardrobe for a while than to waste money on a piece that doesn't work for your style or your life.

HABIT 3: PAY ATTENTION TO DETAILS

Think a white T-shirt is just a white T-shirt? Think again! There are crew necks, V-necks, or boat necks; cap sleeves, raglan sleeves, and half sleeves; A-line fits, straight fits, slim fits, or relaxed fits; cotton, linen, or synthetic fibers. And all these tiny details matter. These details can mean the difference between an all-American Ivy League style and edgy boho-chic. Because in combination, they give a garment personality and a very specific look.

Your ability to create outfits that are in tune with your personal style is completely dependent on how well each individual garment in your wardrobe reflects that style. And that's why training yourself to pay attention to details like the fit, fabric composition, or neckline of an item is such an important step toward building a better wardrobe.

Let's say you want to add a new basic to your wardrobe: a pair of jeans in a dark wash. Now, instead of going with the first pair of dark-wash jeans you find in your size, stop and have a closer look. What fit style do these jeans have? Are they slim, straight, boyfriend, or skinny? Would that fit work well with the rest of your wardrobe, and is it in line with your overall style? Do you like the material? Does it work with the overall look you are going for? What about the rise, the fading, and the placement of the pockets? Are they comfortable to move in?

At the beginning, while your personal style is still a work in progress, paying attention to every detail of a garment might feel a little cumbersome. But once you feel confident about your style and know exactly what types of pieces you need to express it, you'll be able to develop rules of thumb (like you did on page 76) that will speed up the process. For example, it took me a while to figure out that I'm not a fan of scoop necklines or really any neckline that's neither very high nor very low. But now that I know that, I can just go straight to my trusty crew necks or deep V's while I'm out shopping, and it doesn't take any extra time at all.

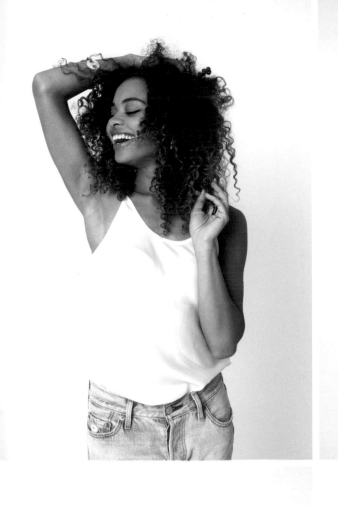
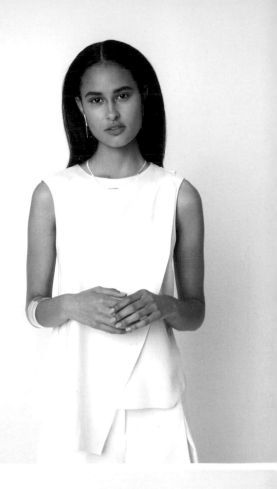
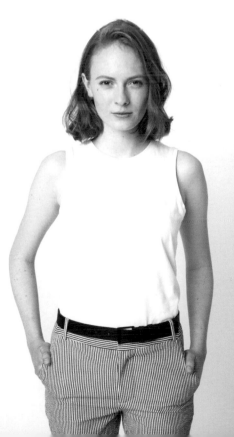
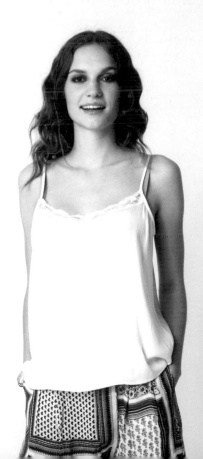

17/

Decision time: When to buy and when to keep looking

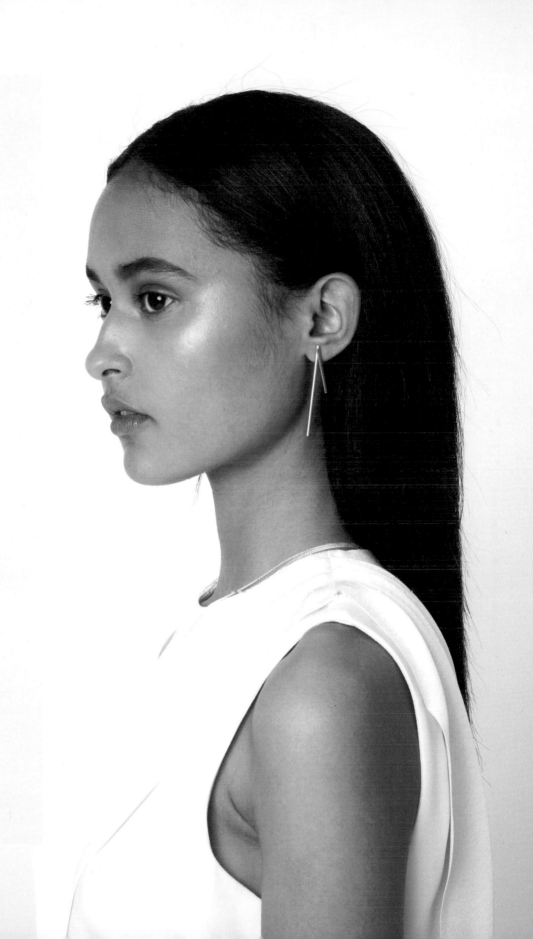

Here's an easy way to make better purchasing decisions, and thirteen questions to ask yourself before you spend your money.

Nobody likes dressing rooms: the lighting is terrible, and you're crammed into a tiny space with a mountain of clothes and a long line of fellow shoppers standing just behind the curtain, waiting for you to hurry up and take your pick already. Making smart purchasing decisions under those circumstances is definitely no easy feat, even if you took the time to write a detailed shopping list beforehand.

When I first started to make a conscious effort to shift my approach to shopping, dressing rooms were always my downfall. I would enter a store with a clear idea of what I needed to buy and every intention to spend money only on things that truly fit my style, my body, and my wardrobe. But once I had tried on a couple of things and it came to making a final decision, I would slip up and forget all about my good intentions.

Sometimes, if I really loved a novel detail, the overall style, or the color of a piece, I'd get so excited that I would just head straight to the cash register, ignoring all practical considerations or the fact that I already had several other pieces just like it hanging in my closet. Sometimes, if the store had a sale going on, I would convince myself that, in exchange for a 20 percent discount, it's okay if that top feels a little scratchy or the straps dig into my shoulders. And sometimes, I would also just be so exhausted after a long day of shopping that I would simply settle for a piece that I knew wasn't ideal, just to be able to cross it off my list.

At first I felt really discouraged by my apparent inability to stick to my shopping resolutions, but then I remembered something I had learned in a social psychology class: humans are pretty terrible at making decisions under pressure. We ignore crucial pieces of information, get hung up on irrelevant details, and overemphasize certain things just to reach a conclusion.

Having to make a decision while stuck in a tiny compartment in various states of undress definitely classifies as an under-pressure situation. And I'm not just talking about time pressure (not wanting to be rude by taking up the room for too long), but also an internal pressure not to leave empty-handed. Because after you've already invested all that time and effort to come to the store and try everything on, of course you'd rather not leave without having anything to show for it.

Automating the process

The hands-down best way to escape that feeling of being under pressure and improve your decision making when it comes to buying pieces for your wardrobe is to simply automate the entire process.

> Put together a little checklist of everything you want to consider before buying something new, from the overall style to its quality and price point, and then just run through it point by point.

Working with a checklist like that has two major advantages:

1. It helps you make sure you have really considered a piece from all angles. Under pressure, it's so easy to cut corners and focus exclusively on the visual characteristics of a piece and ignore things like the fit, fabric, or quality, all of which could be potential deal breakers.
2. It helps take some of the emotion out of the decision and makes it more objective and thereby less susceptible to outside pressure or your random mood.

In this chapter, you'll find a blueprint for such a process that you can tweak to your own needs or use as is. The process consists of thirteen questions in total that will help you assess a potential new wardrobe addition from the following five different perspectives.

STYLE

How well does this piece reflect your personal style?

FUNCTION

How well does this piece fit into the structure of your wardrobe, and how versatile is it?

QUALITY

What's its quality like, from both a subjective (fit and comfort level) and objective point (construction, fabric, and durability) of view?

BUDGET

Is this the best use of your budget right now?

GUT

Do you really love this piece and are you excited to wear it?

Yes, going through all these questions takes a little more effort than just making a rash decision, but remember that being thorough before you buy something and spending a few extra minutes is still a lot easier and less stressful than having to deal with the various frustrations of bad buys later on.

Style

DOES THIS PIECE REFLECT MY PERSONAL STYLE?

As a very first step, give any garment you spot online or on a rack while out shopping a quick glance over to check whether it fits in with the overall direction you have in mind for your wardrobe. Ask yourself: Would this piece help you create that aesthetic or distract from it? Would it fit into the mood board you created to summarize your style or would it stick out like a sore thumb? What about its individual components, like the fabric, details, cut, and colors: are they in line with the style preferences you included in your style profile?

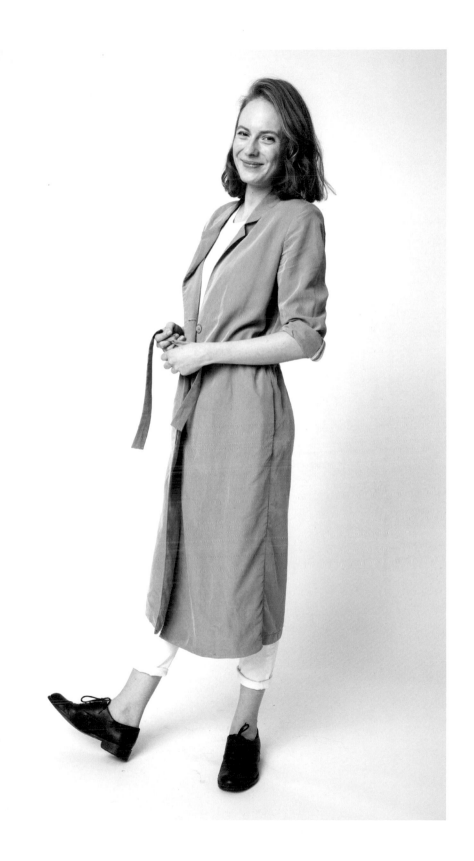

DO I LIKE HOW IT LOOKS ON MY BODY?

There will always be some pieces that you love in theory or on other people, but not so much on yourself. And that's okay. If an item looks gorgeous on the rack or the model but somehow "off" on you, just move on and find a better alternative.

Function

CAN I THINK OF A CLEAR ROLE FOR THIS ITEM WITHIN MY WARDROBE?

To be functional and give you lots of outfit options to choose from, your wardrobe needs to be more than just a random collection of stand-alone pieces. Every new piece you add should be a part of an overall strategy and you should be able to clearly pinpoint what role a new garment would play within your wardrobe.

Would you wear it as a key piece, a statement piece, or a basic? And would it actually work with the clothes you already have in your closet that you usually pair with those items? Run through a few different outfits in your head. For example, If you're thinking about buying an embellished statement top that you would want to pair with your basics, imagine how it would look with the dark-wash jeans and simple skirts you already own.

If you get a feeling the garment wouldn't work well in the role you had in mind for it, chances are it wouldn't fit in well with the rest of your wardrobe and you would have to work around it more than anything.

DOES IT WORK WITH MY LIFESTYLE?

There's no point in wasting money on clothes you would rarely, if ever, get the opportunity to wear. Your wardrobe should support your life as is. So, make sure you know exactly what types of activities or occasions for which you would wear a potential new wardrobe addition. Would you wear it during the day, for work, or to go out at night?

And would the individual components of the piece (the fabric, heel height, or silhouette) actually work well for those activities? Try to come up with a few real-life scenarios, like "drinks with friends" or "running errands on the weekend," to help you spot any obvious mismatches between the qualities of your piece and an activity.

IS IT MIXABLE?

If you want a versatile wardrobe that will give you a ton of different options, each piece should be as mixable as possible. If during any of the previous questions you notice that your piece really works only as part of one or two outfits, it might not be a good investment, especially if you had planned on using it as a basic or a key piece.

You can also evaluate the mixability of a piece by comparing it to your outfit formulas and color palette. As you already know, the goal isn't to wear only shades from your color palette, just like not everything in your wardrobe needs to be a part of one of your outfit formulas. But every piece you buy should at least work with some of the colors in your palette, so you'll have something to wear it with. And if a piece fits right into one of your go-to looks, that's a good indicator you'll get a lot of wears out it.

Quality

DOES IT FIT WELL AND IS IT COMFORTABLE?

No matter whether you are buying a blazer, a pair of pants, or a basic tank top, a great fit is a nonnegotiable. Garments should follow the natural curves of your body and allow you to move freely. Nothing should bulge, pucker, billow, or wrinkle. Whether a piece ticks all these boxes really isn't something you can accurately assess by looking at a picture online. So if you haven't done so yet, now is the time to order the item in question or try it on at a store. Use the essential two-step fit check described on page 244 to evaluate your piece from all angles. Be ruthless here: an item that's an inch outside of your style concept is something you can work with, but a bad fit is a deal breaker.

IS THE GARMENT WELL-CONSTRUCTED AND MADE FROM A HIGH-QUALITY MATERIAL?

A great fit and high comfort level are usually already good indicators for the overall quality of the piece. But to make sure your garment is durable and won't fall apart after a couple of washes, take a minute to also check out the construction and craftsmanship of the piece: Do the seams look neat and sturdy? Does the fabric look tightly woven and strong or flimsy and see-through? Can you see any pills, stray threads, or loose stitches? For more info on how to assess the quality of a piece, refer to chapter 19: Assessing garment quality (page 222).

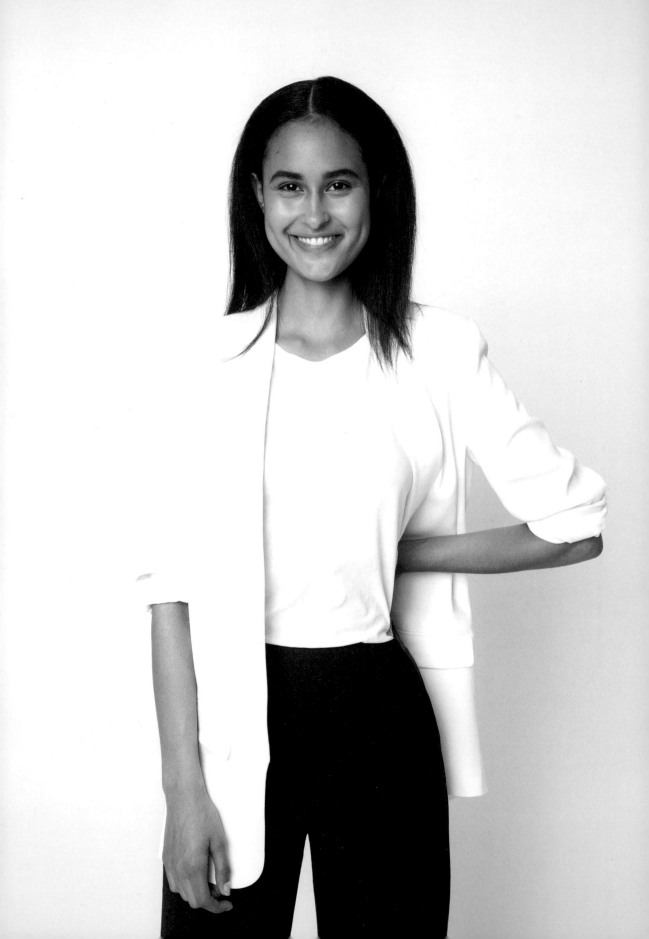

AM I PREPARED TO PROPERLY TAKE CARE OF THIS ITEM?

Never forget to look at the care label of a potential new wardrobe addition. Will you be able to just throw it in with the rest of your laundry or does it need special treatment? Are you willing to have the piece dry cleaned regularly? Do you hate to iron things? Nothing ruins the look and lifespan of a garment faster than improper care, so make sure you are willing and realistically able to give your item what it needs in the long run, whether that means handwashing, ironing, or taking it to the dry cleaner.

Budget

WILL THIS PIECE FILL A GAP IN MY WARDROBE OR ONLY ADD TO AN ALREADY OVERREPRESENTED AREA?

Unless you have an unlimited budget and endless closet space, you have to prioritize certain purchases over others, at least in the short-term. A quick first way to check whether a piece would be a good use of your budget is to simply think about how well-represented that category of items currently is in your wardrobe.

Not even the most gorgeous, high quality maxi dress is worth buying if you already have ten similar ones hanging in your closet. If you have already built up a solid foundation of wardrobe essentials, feel free to spend your money on things you love but don't technically "need." But until then, focus on closing any gaps in your wardrobe first.

IS BUYING THIS PIECE THE BEST USE OF MY BUDGET, OR WOULD A DIFFERENT ITEM MAKE A BIGGER IMPACT ON MY WARDROBE RIGHT NOW?

If your closet needs a lot of work and you have several pieces on your shopping list that all fill crucial gaps in your wardrobe, try to prioritize pieces that will have the biggest *immediate* impact on your ability to build outfits that reflect your style. For example, instead of buying a gorgeous pair of strappy heels that you would get to wear only twice a month, spend that money on a great jacket that you can wear several times a week and that would tie your whole look together.

DO I WANT TO BUY THIS BECAUSE IT'S ON SALE OR I NEED A PICK-ME-UP, WANT TO CELEBRATE, OR AM JUST PLAIN BORED?

If you are prone to overspending and impulse buys, take a moment to double-check that the sole reason you want to buy this piece is because it will help you express your personal style and fill a gap in your wardrobe. If you even have an inkling that you might just be bored or stressed, put the item on hold and walk away. If you still want the piece once those feelings have passed, you can always go back for it later.

Gut

CAN I THINK OF AT LEAST THREE CONCRETE OUTFITS I COULD CREATE WITH THIS PIECE THAT I WOULD BE EXCITED TO WEAR?

If your piece has made it this far, it would definitely be a great addition to your wardrobe from a practical standpoint. Now, make sure your heart's in it too. If you can come up with at least three outfit combos for the piece that you would put on right now if you could, that's a good sign!

CAN I SEE MYSELF WEARING THIS FOR MANY SEASONS?

To build a great wardrobe, you need a long-term focus. If you can already tell you'll be over the piece by the end of the year, don't waste your money on it. A piece that truly reflects your personal style will be something you'll want to keep and cherish for a long time.

When to Buy and When To Keep Looking Cheat Sheet

Make a copy of this page (or take a picture of it with your phone) and take it with you the next time you go shopping.

Style

1. Does this piece reflect my personal style?

2. Do I like how it looks on my body?

Function

3. Can I think of a clear role for this item within my wardrobe?

4. Does it work with my lifestyle, and do I know exactly which type of activities I could wear it for?

5. Is it mixable?

Quality

6. Does it fit well and is it comfortable?

7. Is the garment well-constructed and made from a high-quality material?

8. Am I prepared to properly take care of this item?

Budget

9. Will this piece fill a gap in my wardrobe or only add to an already overrepresented area?

10. Is buying this piece a good use of my budget, or would a different item make a bigger impact on my wardrobe right now?

11. Do I want to buy this because it's on sale or I need a pick-me-up, want to celebrate, or am just plain bored?

Gut

12. Can I think of at least three concrete outfits I could create with this piece that I would be excited to wear?

13. Can I see myself wearing this for many seasons?

18/
How to stop overspending and make the most of your budget

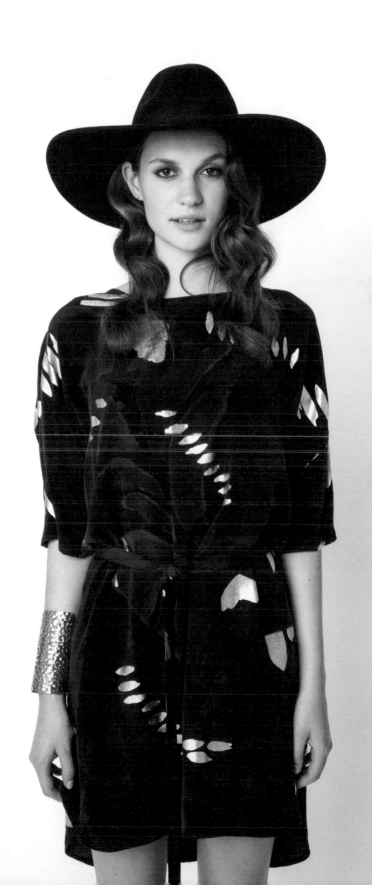

Don't let your spending habits keep you from building your dream wardrobe! Instead, identify your personal triggers for overspending and rethink your approach to shopping the sale section.

How do you spend your money? Do you like to weigh the pros and cons of everything, no matter how tiny the purchase? Do you have a tendency to shop on impulse or when you are stressed or bored? Are you all about finding the best bargains and as a rule won't buy anything that's not on sale? Do you shop for fun or to reward yourself?

Just like your eating habits, your approach to shopping is something you have been cultivating your whole life. And that's why changing it usually requires a good deal of effort and introspection. But it can be done!

This chapter is all about how to make the most of your budget. But by that I do *not* mean how to hunt down the best deals. I'm not much of a fan of bargain hunting, as you probably know by now, and I'll talk more about why that is on pages 220-221. Here's what making the most out of your budget means to me instead:

- Using whatever money you have to spend wisely by prioritizing pieces that will have a big impact on your wardrobe
- *Not* blowing money on random pieces because you are stressed, sad, bored, or want to celebrate

You've already learned how to set priorities and write clear, detailed shopping lists in chapters 16 and 17. Now let's tackle the thoughtful shopper's enemy number one: overspending.

Why we overspend

TO RELIEVE STRESS OR REWARD OURSELVES

Many of us use shopping as a way to manage our emotions: to reduce negative ones and amplify good ones. We reward ourselves with a trip to our favorite store after a big presentation. We shop online after a stressful day at work to relax. We buy stuff we don't need when we're anxious, sad, or frustrated. We use shopping to self-soothe and self-pamper.

We do this because our body has accepted shopping as an efficient way to trigger the release of dopamine in our brain's reward system. We may feel stressed out, but then we enter a shop, browse through all the racks on the lookout for something we like, and when we find it: boom, we feel better, at least for the moment. Over time, that association between buying new stuff and the emotional reward becomes stronger and stronger, until it's turned into a full-blown habit, and we start craving a "fix" whenever we feel particularly bad or good.

Try this instead

If you have a tendency to overspend when you're sad, anxious, or super happy, try these two steps:

1. Analyze your individual triggers for wanting to buy stuff.
2. Figure out a replacement strategy, such as activities you can do instead of shopping.

For example, if you tend to shop online at night after a long day at work, make a list of things you could do instead in the evenings to relax, like taking a bubble bath, calling a friend, curling up on the couch with a book, cuddling your cat, and so on. The key is to make the decision to do something other than shopping before the trigger happens and have everything prepared for that activity, to make it super easy *not* to shop once you are in the habit cycle.

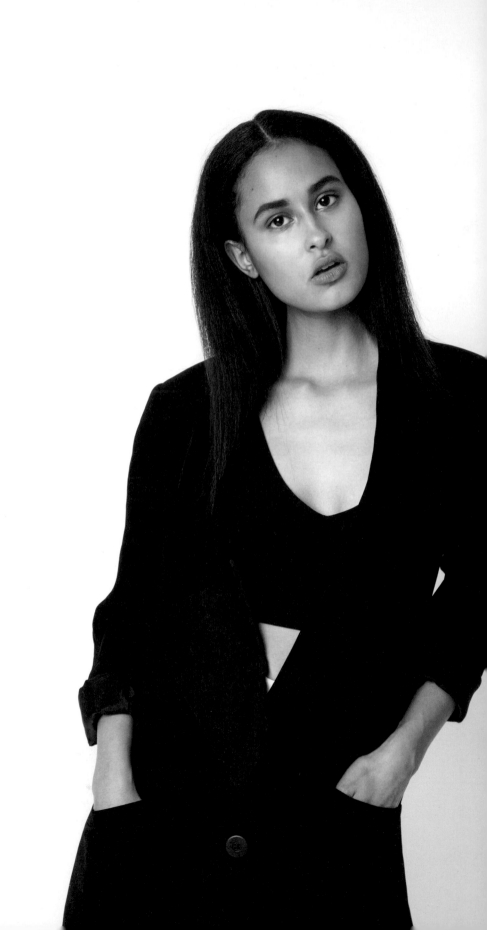

TO HAVE FUN AND PASS THE TIME

For many people, shopping is also just another fun way to spend the afternoon, evening, or weekend—walking through the city (perhaps with a friend or two), browsing through racks and shelves of stuff, the thrill of finding something you love, building outfits in your head, and the anticipation of wearing a new piece for the first time. If you love clothes and see fashion as a way to be creative and express yourself, all these things are fun for you, just like watching a game live at a stadium is fun for a football fan or going to the movies is fun for a cinephile.

Try this instead

If you love fashion but tend to overspend your budget because of it, try to find ways to have fun with fashion and be creative that don't involve buying something. Keep honing your personal style, experiment, find different ways to wear your old favorites. Get into fashion illustration, photography, or any other creative medium. Swap clothes with friends. Or start a blog (on fashion, not shopping)!

OUT OF UNCERTAINTY OR A LACK OF CONFIDENCE

Some people shop too much, not because it's fun or stress relieving for them but to fix a problem. If you are unhappy with your wardrobe or the way you look, buying a new pair of shoes or a beauty product is a way of taking charge and solving the problem. If you think your clothes aren't good, trendy, or chic enough, new stuff will make you feel as if you are making progress, at least for a little while. Of course, adding more and more pieces to an already bursting closet without a clear direction will only make it even more difficult to feel confident about your style and build outfits you feel great in.

Try this instead

Take a step back and do a little soul-searching: do you lack confidence in general or are you just not sure about your personal style? If it's the latter, it's key that you take your time working through the style-defining steps in this book before you tackle your wardrobe and buy new pieces. If it's a confidence issue, focus on building up your self-esteem in other areas of your life first.

 Do you have a tendency to overspend? If so, what is your personal trigger? And what could you do instead of shopping from now on, whenever you feel the urge?

A quick tip to avoid impulse buys

Identifying your personal shopping trigger should immediately help reduce overspending by keeping you out of the shops in the first place. But what if you really do need something specific and have to enter the danger zone (read: the mall, your favorite store, or an online shop)? Here's a super quick and easy tip for those situations: *Delay the purchase!*

Put some time between the impulse and the purchase. If you see something that you like but hadn't planned on buying, put it on hold for a day. If you still love the item the next day, after having had a chance to really think it through, buy it. For shopping online, add the item to a wish list or just save the link.

Go on a shopping fast

In our culture, buying a ton of new stuff every year has become the norm. We are so used to buying new clothes, gadgets, and knickknacks all the time that buying less, repairing what you have instead of immediately replacing it, and putting time and effort into selecting new purchases all seem like foreign concepts. An effective way to reset what you consider normal and gain a new perspective is going on a temporary shopping fast. Don't buy anything for one whole week and see how you feel. Or don't buy anything new for one month except for food and essentials like shampoo and toilet paper. You can also limit your shopping fast to just one specific group of things you're having trouble with, like clothes or beauty products. Throughout your fast, keep a little diary of how you feel so you can later go back to identify your personal triggers for wanting to shop and find replacement activities.

Beware the sale!

Holiday sales, end-of-year sales, coupons, limited editions, store cards: Discounts are the Trojan horses of the retail industry. And learning how to navigate them is one of the best things you can do for your budget and your wardrobe. And, in most instances, by *navigate* I mean *avoid*.

"What? But sales help me save money!" you might say. Do they really, though? Because let's not forget what discounts are: a marketing tool designed to get us to spend *more* money, not less. Price reductions are one of the most reliable sales strategies out there and a surefire way for a brand to increase profit.

Why do discounts work so well? Because they tap right into our inherent fear of scarcity and trigger our instinct to hoard resources whenever we can. We tend to use the price of a product as a marker for its desirability, so when something is reduced, we feel as though by buying it we are making the best possible use of our most-valued resource: money. That coupled with the fact that time-limited discounts create a sense of urgency puts us straight back into hunter-gatherer mode.

And sure, there is nothing wrong with feeling a little extra satisfaction when you find a piece you love that's *also* on sale. The trouble is when the price reduction is the central reason for purchasing, when hunting down the best deals becomes a sport, and when you spend money so you can save money.

> When that happens, we end up with a wardrobe full of pieces that may all have been a bargain but that were still a waste of money.

Because no matter the price, a new piece is worth the money only if you need it, love it, and will wear it. A fifteen-dollar scarf that doesn't work with the rest of your wardrobe is not a good deal, even if it originally cost fifty dollars. And that pair of designer jeans that's just a little too short may come at an almost irresistible 50 percent off right now, but that still doesn't make it a sensible investment if you never end up wearing them.

That's not to say you can't take advantage of sales. The trick is just to make sure you are using discounts only as a secondary factor when shopping. For example, if you are on the market for a new pair of winter boots, go ahead and check the sale sections of your favorite stores to see whether they have a pair that fits your criteria.

Notice how that approach is different from browsing the sales to see whether they might have something you like, or finding something to buy at store X because you still have a coupon. Because, even if you head out with the clear intention to buy only things you need, your hunter-gatherer mode will always find a way to convince you that, at 30 percent off, that black sequinned T-shirt really is too good to pass up because "you can never have too many T-shirts."

The easiest way to prevent that from happening is to make your purchasing decisions independently from the discount. Decide what you want to buy— whether that is a leather jacket, a pencil skirt, or a statement necklace—and then see whether a piece that fits your criteria is available at a discount.

19 / Assessing garment quality: A beginner's guide

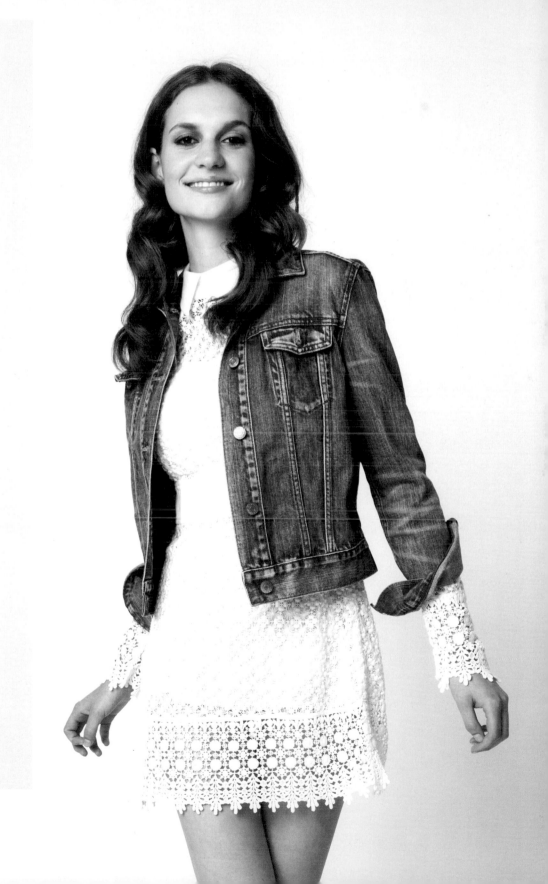

Learn how to evaluate the quality of a potential new wardrobe addition and become a pro at finding high-quality pieces at all price points.

What's the number one prerequisite to building a high-quality wardrobe? Being able to recognize a quality garment when you see one. You need to be able to tell the difference between a durable, well-crafted piece and one that looks pretty on the rack but won't last more than a few washes. You need to know (1) which properties distinguish high-quality garments from low-quality ones and (2) how to spot these properties when you're out shopping.

To help you do just that, this chapter will give you a broad introduction to evaluating the quality of garments based on five key components: fabric, seams, tailoring, lining, and details (such as buttonholes and zippers).

To build a high-quality wardrobe, you need to set priorities. Not every single thing in your closet needs to last twenty years. Not every single sock you own needs to be made from merino wool. Going overboard is never practical, so decide which items you do want to invest a bit more time (and money) in and which you don't mind replacing after a couple of seasons.

What is quality?

Let's go back to basics for a moment: What is quality? And, more specifically, what distinguishes a low-quality garment from a high-quality one?

In general, when we say *quality*, we mean quite a few different but related things: We want our clothes to be durable, to last for more than a couple of seasons. We want sturdy clothes—garments that we can move in without having to worry about ripping seams or popping buttons. We want our clothes to keep the same shape they had when we bought them, and to neither stretch out nor shrink over time. We don't want fabric that pills or fades after wearing or washing it a couple of times. We want our clothes to feel good on the skin so we can enjoy wearing them instead of wanting to take them off as soon as we get home. And lastly, we also want our clothes to *look* like high-quality garments—smooth fabric, neat seams, beautiful detailing—not something that is about to fall apart.

Whether a garment ticks these boxes or not depends on its five key components and how they work together: the fabric, seams, tailoring, lining, and even smaller details like buttons and pockets.

What distinguishes high-quality from low-quality manufacturers are the extra steps they take to make sure a garment not only looks the part now, but also will continue to do so after multiple wears and washes. All of these "extras" take time and money. That's why it's so easy to find pretty pieces at budget stores that end up falling apart after a week: to cut costs, the manufacturer chose to focus on making the garment look good on the hanger instead of its quality, because that is what brings in the sales. Pretty much every shopper makes purchasing decision based on what a garment looks like; only a very few will take the time to assess the seams or the quality of the tailoring.

It's important to note that the quality and the price of an item are not always related. Some types of items are easier to manufacture and get right than others, which is why it is totally possible to find certain well-made items at affordable prices. At the same time, just because an item is very pricy does not always mean that the manufacturer used all that extra money to up the quality of the garment. So get in the habit of inspecting every possible new wardrobe addition up close, regardless of its price and brand.

Fabric

The hands-down most important component of a garment is its fabric. No matter how beautiful the details or how well-crafted the seams are, a garment made from a flimsy, scratchy, or pilling fabric is never a good addition to any wardrobe.

COTTON

Cotton is a super popular fabric for good reason: it's soft, versatile, durable (when high quality), washable, and comparatively affordable. The most important property of cotton is its staple length, that is, the length of the individual fibers comprising the fabric. Fabric made from long cotton fibers is generally considered to be of a higher quality than fabrics made from shorter fibers. Here's why:

- Durability. Longer fibers can be spun into a finer yarn. Fine yarn can be more tightly woven, which makes the resulting fabric stronger and more durable.
- Softness. Another plus of long fibers is that they can be turned into a much softer yarn. The shorter the staple, the more difficult it is to spin the fibers into yarn without having tiny ends of fibers sticking out at all angles. Longer cotton fibers can be closely bound together, which keeps them from going in different directions.
- Breathability. One reason some fabrics are less breathable than others is that they contain tiny air pockets in between the individual threads that create thermal insulation. Cotton made from long, finely spun fibers can be very tightly woven to eliminate air pockets and that uncomfortable, sweaty feeling that we tend to associate with low breathability.

Here's how to estimate whether a cotton garment was made with long-staple fibers or not:

- Touch it! Even cotton fabric that is sturdy, thick, or even stiff should feel soft on the skin. If it doesn't, it was probably made with shorter fibers and will be less durable in the long run.
- It's free of pills. Cotton is generally not as prone to pilling as other fabrics, so if you already see a trace of pilling on a new garment, move on!
- Check the density of the fabric by holding it up to the light. Even if it is very fine, the fabric should not be transparent. If the fabric lets through a lot of light, it's a sign that it is not very dense and therefore will not be very durable.
- Cotton needs to be spun, so look closely at the threads that make up the fabric. There should be no gaps or size differences between the individual threads. All you should see up close is a regular pattern of smooth rows.
- Cotton is an especially good choice when you are shopping at low-end/ budget stores. Some fabrics are hard to get right at the lower end of the price range, but since cotton is comparatively cheap to produce, you should be able to find cotton items that are affordable *and* well made.

LINEN

Linen is made from flax fibers that are naturally smooth but not very elastic. It's a great fabric for summer, because it is breathable, dries fast, has a cooling effect, and is lint resistant. In general, there are fewer quality differences with linen than with cotton, and if a garment already has a high linen content, then that is a good sign. Here are a few more things to look out for when shopping for linen items:

- Make sure the linen feels comfortable on the skin. Linen is not a soft garment by nature, but if it actually feels scratchy or rough, short/low-quality fibers were probably used, which come with all the same disadvantages as short cotton fibers (see page 226).

- The one downside to linen is that it is not very elastic (therefore it wrinkles easily) and will eventually rip if it is constantly folded in the same spot. Before you buy, make sure that the linen does not already contain any small permanent creases that can't be smoothed out. These are likely a sign of a style or cut that creates strong natural folds when you move, and these will only become more pronounced with regular wear. Also, think about whether the item will still look okay when it's a little wrinkled at the end of the day.

- Do not worry about slubs, those tiny, random knots along the yarn of the linen. These are almost always intentionally included in order to keep the integrity of the fibers intact and also add that special natural linen texture. It's also okay if there are no slubs: very fine linen is usually slub-free because it was created from a very fine thread made from fibers of a consistent diameter.

- Always check the care instructions before you buy a linen piece. Linen is very prone to shrinking, and many linen garments can only be dry cleaned or washed in cold water.

WOOL

The quality of wool can generally be determined by the quality of the individual wool fibers that make up the fabric. These in turn depend on the breed of animals that produced them, their diet and stress levels, and how the fibers were handled during the manufacturing process.

Here are some tips for assessing wool:

- Check for any manufacturing faults: the knitting should be consistent and there should not be any knots, loose strands, holes, or gaps between the individual threads of the fabric. One reason for fiber breakage when it comes to wool is that the animal the fiber came from was stressed or malnourished, resulting in a weak or brittle fiber. If you can already see broken fibers on a new garment, chances are they would only multiply with regular wear.

- Pilling is created when individual fibers come loose and eventually curl up into tiny balls. Wool pills easily, although higher-quality variants will be more tightly woven to prevent fibers from becoming loose in the first place. If you want a wool item that pills as little as possible, choose one with a very dense, finely knitted material. And if there aren't any pills on the garment when you try it on (not even on the collar, cuffs, or inner thighs), the item gets a major thumbs-up.

- Wool fabric should be elastic. It should bounce back immediately when you pull it and not stay stretched out.

- Unless it's a part of the design of an item, you should generally not be able to see through the weave. A high-quality wool garment will be tightly woven and dense, without any gaps in between the individual threads.

- In general, fabric made from fine wool fibers will be softer than thicker fibers; however, depending on the item you are looking for, you may prefer a sturdier, coarser type of fabric, even if it is a little scratchy (for outerwear for example). Before you buy a wool item, make sure you test what it feels like, not just on your hands but also on places where your skin is more sensitive, like the inside of your arm, to make sure you like it. Also note that some types of wools are naturally softer than others—for example, cashmere is much softer than mohair—so the softness of a wool item does not necessarily speak for its quality.

DENIM

The quality of denim depends mainly on the quality of the cotton used to create it and how it was woven. Another important property is the stitching on the item (that is not technically a fabric property, but since it's very denim-specific I want to mention some points about that here). The wash of the final piece is what really tends to drive the price of denim up, but that is not so much a question of quality but of added labor and production costs. Here are some more pointers for assessing the quality of denim pieces:

- Denim made from high-quality cotton feels soft and even, as if it's a little moist.

- Denim should never feel thin and flimsy or so stiff and heavy that you can't move (unless it is a raw, unwashed piece), but anything in between is fine and a matter of personal choice. If you want to go for a thinner fabric, make sure the yarns are tightly woven and the fabric feels strong and dense, so it won't tear easily.

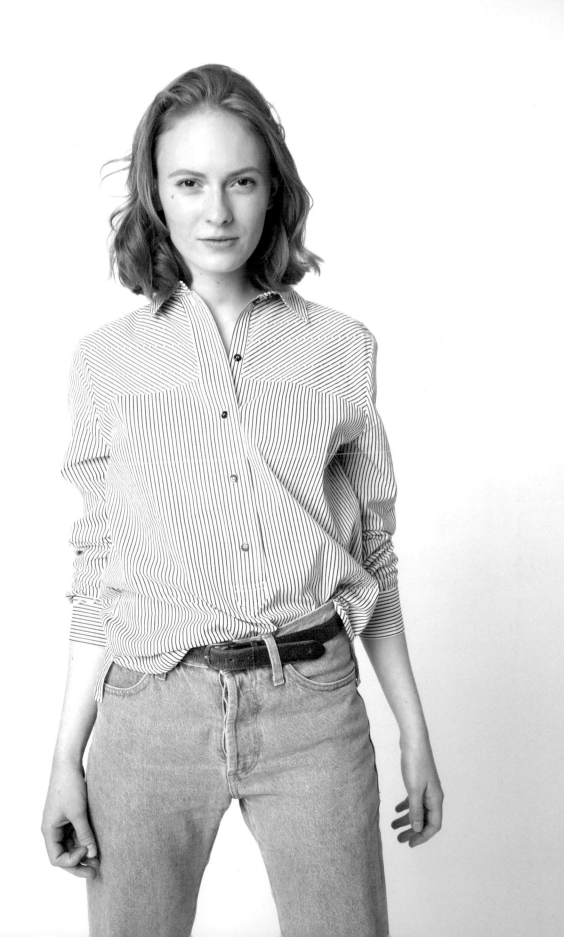

- When you are buying denim secondhand, always check the inner thighs for rubbing. If there is a lot of visible wear and tear, chances are the quality of the denim fabric is low.

- Since denim is a very heavy fabric, strong seams that won't split or unravel under stress are super important. As a first step, try stretching the denim piece at different places along the seams. If the threads of the seams pull apart, not so good. Then check the stitching. High-quality denim manufacturers will usually use either double stitching (two rows of stitching next to each other) or chain stitching (looped stitches that look like links of chain). As long as the thread is very thick, a single row of stitches is also okay, but make sure you do the stretching test in that case.

- Another way to assess the quality of a pair of denim jeans is to look at how the side seams were done. The cheapest, easiest way is to sew the two pieces of fabric together, then cut off the excess. This method leaves a bump along the inner side of your leg. High-quality manufacturers instead take the extra step to first sew the edges of each side before they sew them together and press the seam flat for a streamlined outline.

LEATHER

Leather is not technically a fabric but a material. The quality of a leather piece mainly depends on what type of "grain" it has. Full-grain leather is generally considered the highest-quality type and refers to leather that has not been sanded, buffed, or corrected to retain the skin's natural fiber strength and durability. Top-grain (also called corrected grain) and split grain leather have been more heavily processed (the top layer of the skin is usually removed) and are therefore not as durable as full-grain leather; they also won't develop that coveted natural patina of high-quality leather over time. Here are some more notes on leather quality:

- Look closely at the tiny grains on the fabric. Do they look natural or printed? Brands that use corrected leather will sometimes print marks back onto the sanded leather to add authenticity. Up close these printed grains will look much more uniform than full-grain leather—won't contain any of the natural imperfections that full-grain leather would have from the animal from which it came.

- A major downside of leather is that it can be permanently creased. When you buy a new piece, make sure it does not already have any scratch marks. On unworn pieces, those usually signify that the leather is either brittle or very high maintenance.

- Check how the individual pieces of leather are attached. Were they sewn together or glued? Stitching takes longer than gluing and is therefore more expensive for brands, but it creates a stronger hold between the pieces. Any visible remains of glue are a definite no-go.

VEGAN LEATHER

A great alternative to real leather is faux (or vegan) leather, which usually consists of a polyurethane coating on a fibrous layer. High-quality faux leather can be just as durable as real leather, is generally more affordable and easier to maintain, won't lighten as much in the sun, and doesn't involve the death of animals.

- Just like real leather, faux leather should feel supple, not have any obvious scratch marks, and the individual parts of the item should be sewn rather than glued together.
- Low-quality faux leather will often have an obvious plasticky, shiny look to it; higher quality pieces are almost indistinguishable from animal leather, at least to nonexperts.
- So, avoid shiny; go for soft and supple and, when in doubt, know that thicker tends to be better. Faux leather can be lightweight, but it should never feel thin or flimsy.

SYNTHETICS: IS NATURAL ALWAYS BETTER?

The short answer is no. Although many people will consider even small amounts of manufactured fibers in a fabric's composition a negative, synthetic or semisynthetic fibers do have their advantages and can make a great alternative or addition to natural fibers. Here's why:

- For starters, there is a huge difference between synthetic materials (usually polyester or viscose) that are commonly used by budget fashion brands and the high-quality synthetic materials used by designers or higher-quality brands. In the fast-fashion industry, synthetic materials are often used to *replace* natural fibers. It's about cutting costs, so these types of synthetic fibers typically won't have a high quality and are mainly chosen for their resemblance to natural materials, their price, or their look. On the other end of the spectrum there is the designer who chooses a synthetic material over a natural one for its specific properties (it's particularly lightweight, the way it drapes, its texture), in order to enhance the final garment. Many designers and brands specifically formulate fabrics to get the exact type that's right for their design or to improve things like breathability and other functional properties.

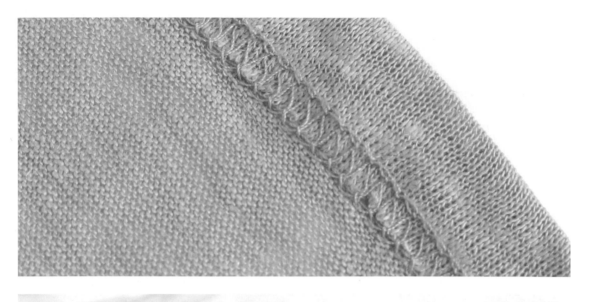

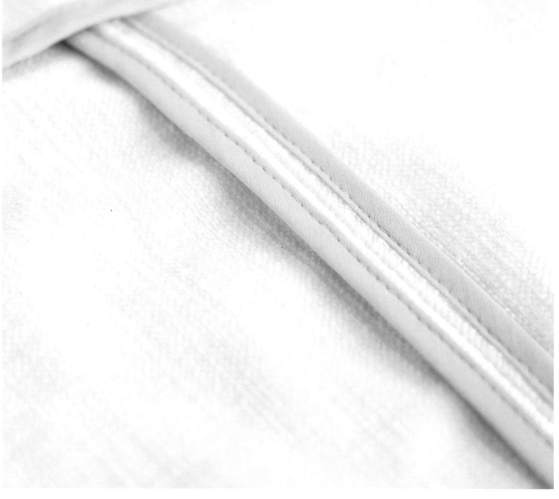

- Oftentimes, a small amount of synthetic fiber improves the fit of an otherwise natural fabric. Spandex, polyester, or Lycra especially, mix well with cottons or wools to add stretch and elasticity and make sure the garment keeps its shape after washing. For fitted items that you want to curve around your body (such as jeans or T-shirts), look for a fabric composition that includes about 2 to 5 percent of a stretchy synthetic material.
- Synthetic fibers are often the best choice for activewear because they are lightweight, super stretchy (and therefore formfitting without being restricting), dry fast, or are able to wick sweat away from the skin.

Seams

The seams of a garment are generally a fail-proof indicator of its quality, because, although they are hugely important for the durability and shape of a garment, the average shopper will typically pay little attention to them. That's why low-budget manufacturers like to save money and time by skipping the extra seam work it takes to turn a garment from something that holds up and looks fine on the rack into a durable garment that will retain its shape and structure over time. Here are a few ways to check the quality of the seams on a garment

GENERAL PROPERTIES
- First, look over the main seams of the item. Are they straight or crooked, neat or messy? Stray threads, loose stitches, or areas that have been stitched over multiple times are all bad signs. There should also not be any obvious needle holes in the seams. A needle that is too large for the fabric, a basic manufacturing mistake that weakens the seam over time, likely created these. To check the strength of the seam, try pulling on the fabric a little on either side. If the seam separates, it was poorly manufactured.
- Second, make sure that all seams on the fabric lie completely flat without puckering. The seams of a garment should never break up its silhouette and should "seamlessly" integrate into the piece.
- Third, if a garment is patterned, check whether the patterns line up at the seams. High-quality brands will make sure a patterned garment looks as though it consists of one piece of fabric; low-quality brands will usually skip that extra step to save money.

TYPES OF SEAMS

Another indicator of quality is the *type* of seams the manufacturer used to connect the individual pieces of fabric. As a rule of thumb, you want neat, secure, reinforced seams instead of a few flimsy stitches. However, depending on the item and also the role of the seam within the fabric, you'll need to look out for slightly different things:

- Start with the inside of the garment. A very common way to sew seams is to serge them. A serged seam has a distinct zigzag pattern and is one of the fastest, cheapest ways to seam a garment. Now, even though serged seams are not particularly strong, they are completely fine for finishing edges on garments like T-shirts and lightweight shirts, particularly when the edge is folded under first. What they are no good for is load-bearing seams, that is, any seam that connects two pieces of fabrics, like side seams on trousers, shoulder seams, and also the hemlines of items made from heavier fabrics. Because load-bearing seams are under constant tension, they should be created using a more secure method, such as using double stitches (two rows of stitches close to each other), French seams (the edges of each piece of fabric are folded under and then sewn together), or bound seams (the edges are each folded under and then enclosed in a strip of fabric).

- Now, on to the outside of the garment. In general, high-quality manufacturers will want to hide outer seams as much as possible (unless they are a part of the design). Load-bearing seams should all be neat, secure (do the pulling test), and not too noticeable. A stable, secure hemline is also crucial for the shape of a piece, so finish off your seam inspection by checking out the lower edge of the piece. The hemlines of lower-quality garments will usually just be folded under and sewn in place. In that case you would be able to clearly see a line of stitches on the outside and serged zigzag lines on the inside. Like I said above, this type of seam is fine for lightweight items, but for things like jackets, trousers, and skirts, which depend on a strong hemline to retain their shape, you are better off with a bound seam or an invisible finish (which uses a blind hem stitch to attach the hemline to the garment and is barely visible from the outside).

Tailoring

Our bodies are not two-dimensional; that's why almost every garment needs a little tailoring to make it fit the contours of our shape. To what extent a brand takes the extra time to do this says a lot about the overall quality of its collection. Now, more than any other point in this chapter, tailoring obviously has a strong individual component. Although a number of things are universal (there should always be a back seam in jackets, for example), a major portion of what "good tailoring" means to you will depend on your body's proportions. What works for you might not work on your friend and vice versa, so make sure you always assess the tailoring of a garment from both an objective (best practices of tailoring) *and* a subjective (whether it works for your body) perspective. Chapter 20 is dedicated to that subjective perspective, to assessing how well a piece fits the individual contours of your body. In this section, we'll look at a few objective properties of good tailoring:

- Items like shirts, blouses, jackets, and nonstretchy dresses and tops should have darts on the front and under the bust to pull in the bottom of the item to your waist and make sure the fabric underneath the bustline does not bulge or hang.
- The seams on the shoulders of jackets and tailored tops should be reinforced to prevent them from becoming stretched out over time.
- Something that many budget manufacturers skip is a seam down the center of the back. Your back is not flat, which is why a square piece of fabric will never look as good as a piece with at least one if not multiple back seams that follow the curve of your back. Stretchy tops do not necessarily need a back seam, but definitely look for one on jackets and coats.
- Many high-quality shirts and blouses have a shoulder yoke, which is an extra piece of fabric that sits on your shoulders and around the neckline, connecting the front and back piece of the shirt. A shoulder yoke is not a must, but it does allow for a neater fit around the shoulders and a smoother drape across the front and back.
- Another way cheaper brands save money is by skipping facings and interfacings. An interfacing is an extra piece of fabric sewn in between the outer layer and the lining of a piece to support its structure and keep it from stretching out, for example along the shoulders or button placket. The only way to figure out whether a garment includes an interfacing is to feel it with your hands. A facing is a piece of fabric that encloses the raw edges inside a garment opening (such as around the waistband, sleeve opening, neckline, or collar) to protect the seams and help the garment keep its shape.

Lining

- Any garment with a high-quality lining should get major bonus points! Linings are great for a lot of reasons: they give the garment a neater finish on the inside by hiding (and protecting) seams, interfacings, padding, and all that stuff; they add an extra layer of warmth; and they protect the outer shell of the garment from skin oils and sweat, which greatly prolongs the lifespan of the piece. They also allow you to slip more easily into the garment, which reduces the tension on the outer layer and keeps the fabric from becoming baggy or stretched out. For items like fitted skirts, a lining also greatly improves fit because it prevents the outer fabric from clinging to your thighs and thereby creates a more streamlined silhouette.

- Linings are a must for some types of garments, but not all of them. Items that should be lined include anything that is very constructed or tailored, difficult to clean, or delicate. Think lighter, see-through fabrics as well as jackets, coats, structured dresses, loosely woven fabrics, suedes, leathers, knits, and tailored skirts.

- Assess the fabric of the lining as you would any other fabric and make sure you like how it feels on your skin. In general, linings should be made from a thicker, sturdier material that is antistatic. Whether you prefer cotton, satin, or a wool mix is up to you, but always make sure that the lining has the same care code as the upper fabric, otherwise getting it cleaned is going to be a huge hassle. On many pieces from more affordable brands, you'll often find linings made from acetate, a synthetic fabric that is made from wood pulp. Acetate is soft, biodegradable, absorbs moisture, and drapes well without clinging to your skin, which makes it a good lining fabric. Unfortuately, it also tends to shrink in the wash and should therefore be dry-cleaned, which makes "affordable" pieces with an acetate lining not so affordable in the long run.

Details

Reinforced buttonholes, flat zippers, real pockets: The finishing touches of a garment are telltale signs of its overall quality. Here's how to inspect the buttons, zippers, pockets, and label of a potentional new wardrobe addition.

BUTTONS AND ZIPPERS

- Check that the buttons are spaced out evenly and secured by multiple threads to keep them in place. There should also be at least one extra button included with every item. High-quality labels will usually attach these to the care label or the hemline.

- Even more important than the buttons themselves are the buttonholes, which should always be reinforced to keep the button from pulling on the fabric unevenly or even ripping through. Ideally, buttonholes should be bound or reinforced by very densely stitched thread. You should not be able to see any raw edges of the fabric through the stitching.

- Buttonholes on jackets and cardigans (or any item that depends on a clean silhouette) should be of the "keyhole" variety, which means that they include a round hole on one side. This allows the button to sit comfortably in the buttonhole without distorting the fabric.
- Always assess the quality of a garment's zipper while you are wearing it; that way you will get a better idea of how the zipper holds up under pressure. Make sure it moves smoothly and lies flat against your body, without puckering. The zipper should also completely lock at the top and not move down if you pull on the sides a little bit.

POCKETS

- High-quality jackets should have real pockets with an adequate length. On fitted or very tailored pieces, pockets may be closed by a line of stitches to keep the silhouette smooth. That allows you to decide whether you would like to use them (by opening the stitches) or not. Another thing to look out for when inspecting pockets is whether the opening is reinforced by a line of neat stitches.

LABELS

- In general, brands that care about the comfort of their garments will use woven, not printed, labels, and place them somewhere it won't feel uncomfortable to the wearer. Avoid anything with a huge, obnoxious plastic label. Even though they can be cut off, it's a pain to remove them completely without tearing the fabric or leaving a tiny but itchy remainder.

20/
Practical pointers for finding clothes that fit well

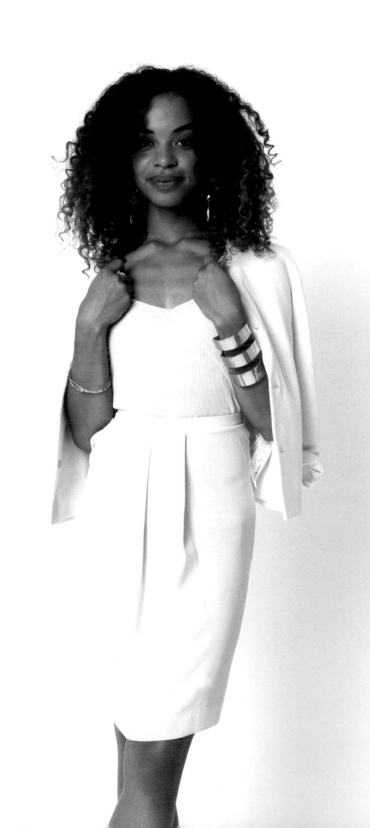

Finding great-fitting clothes doesn't have to be so hard. Use this two-step method to instantly assess the fit of a potential new piece. Plus, learn thirty easy fixes to common fit problems.

Life is too short for uncomfortable clothes.

The sizing across brands is all over the place. We all know that. We've all heard of vanity sizing; we know that what it says on the tag is nothing but an arbitrary number. And just because you are size 6 at one store doesn't mean you can't very well be anything from a size 0 to a size 10 at another store.

If a great fit was just about picking the right size, finding clothes would be easy, and all I'd have to say in this chapter about fit would be, just try on a bunch of different sizes—one of them is going to fit! But it's not quite as easy as that. Because the *size* of your body is just one of two factors that determine how well a garment will fit you. What's the other one? Your *proportions*.

Your proportions include everything from the width of your shoulders and rib cage to the length of your legs and arms and the curve of your waist. Your proportions may be similar to those of another person, but they won't be exactly the same. And sure, we may not be talking about more than a quarter of an inch here or there, but when it comes to a great fit, that extra quarter of an inch makes a big difference.

Finding clothes that match your body's size and proportions is no easy feat. Most people, except for a lucky few, can't just pick out whatever from a rail of clothes and expect a great fit. Our bodies are too unique and complex for that. A little trial and error is inevitable. But that doesn't mean you have to spend hours in dressing rooms just to find a single good pair of jeans.

Here's how to speed up that process: learn how to spot common fit issues and their causes.

That way, instead of blindly trying on a bunch of stuff in the hopes of eventually hitting a jackpot, you can try on just one or two pairs, assess it based on a clear set of criteria, and figure out what the problem is. Based on that, you can then decide your next step—when a piece doesn't fit, you have four options:

1. Try a different size.
2. Try a different style or silhouette if available (for example, a lower-waisted pair of jeans).
3. Have it tailored (more about that on page 245).
4. Skip that piece entirely (when it's poorly constructed, does not work with your proportions, cannot be altered, or isn't worth having altered).

On the next few pages you'll learn all about the most common fit problems, their causes, and how to fix them (using one of the four options above).

As a first step though, you need to know what to look for.

What do good and bad fits look like?

A piece with a **good fit**
- hangs on your body just as the designer intended it to
- feels comfortable and allows you to move freely
- stays put without having to be readjusted

A piece with a **bad fit**
- looks distorted and may be too tight in some places but too loose in others
- digs into your skin, feels uncomfortably tight, and restricts your movement
- slips down, pulls, gaps, wrinkles, or bunches up as you move and needs to be constantly tucked back into place

Often, solving a fit issue is as easy as moving up or down a size. If a coat bunches at the shoulders and makes you look like the Hulk, it may simply be

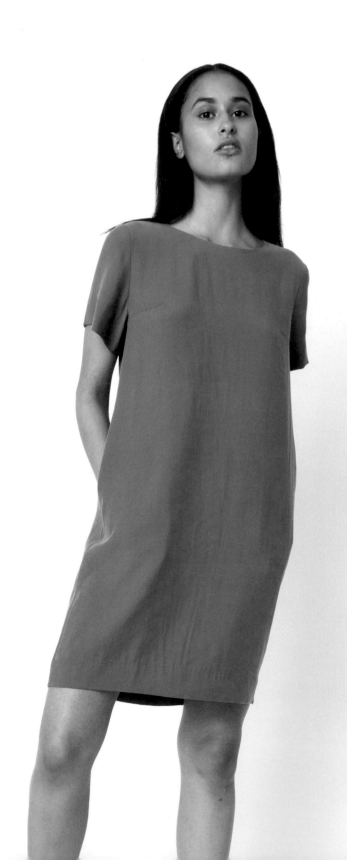

too big for you. If a skirt stretches and wrinkles across the top of your thighs and cuts into your stomach, grab one size up and see if that improves things.

But sometimes, switching sizes fixes one issue but creates another, and that's where it gets a littler tricker. If you are busty, a bigger-size blazer may allow you to button it up, but not without simultaneously hanging off you like a tent from the waist down. And size 29 jeans may accommodate your butt and thighs better than a size 28, but now the waistband is free-floating an inch away from your actual waist, and when you bend over your backside is on full display.

In that case, size isn't the issue. It's the basic construction of the garment.

There are two reasons why a piece may not fit your body, no matter what size you try on.

THE PIECE IS BADLY CONSTRUCTED IN GENERAL

Strange proportions and poorly placed darts, zippers, and armholes: These are all basic manufacturing issues that happen when a brand does not take the time to make sure their pieces are properly tailored, functional, and comfortable. If you suspect a piece might not be well-constructed, just move on. A crafty tailor might be able to fix some basic construction mistakes, but it's usually not worth it.

YOUR BODY'S PROPORTIONS DON'T MATCH THOSE OF THE BRAND'S FIT MODEL

Most brands employ fit models to create their patterns and optimize the fit of their pieces. Besides a ton of patience, fit models must also have proportions that are as close as possible to "average" for their particular size. And in general, that approach is a good one, because it means that the clothes are designed for real bodies (as opposed to mannequins) and the final collection will fit the biggest possible number of people. The trouble is that brands have different views about what they consider to be "average." One brand may design its clothes based on a model with slightly broader shoulders, another on a model that's a little more pear-shaped. And again, these differences are tiny but they matter.

The essential two-step fit check

Here's how to assess the fit of a potential new wardrobe addition in two easy steps.

STEP 1: MIRROR CHECK

Try on your piece in front of a full-length mirror and inspect it top to bottom. Does it look as it should? Or could your crop top be mistaken for a baggy tank top? Is there any creasing, pulling on the seams, or sagging? Pay special attention to the shoulders of tops, jackets, and dresses and the waistband and crotch area of pants and skirts. Does the waistband fit snugly around your body? Or is it too tight, loose, or unsupportive?

✗ If you spot any issues, refer to the next few pages for pointers on what to try on next and whether to get this piece tailored or drop it entirely.

✓ If you didn't spot any issues, your piece has passed the mirror check. Yay! On to step 2.

STEP 2: MOVEMENT CHECK

Pants that slip down a good two inches (resulting in the dreaded "saggy-butt syndrome"), blazers that give you T-rex arms, and skirts that spin around your waist as soon as you take a step—some fit issues become apparent only when you move.

Check how your piece feels and looks during these four basic movements:

1. Hug someone (or pretend to).
2. Sit down.
3. Walk.
4. Bend over (as if your were tying your shoes).

If you like, you can also do some lunges or a little chicken dance. If you are trying on shoes, walk across the room a couple of times.

✗ The piece feels too tight in the shoulders when you raise your arms? You can hardly breathe when you sit down in those pants? Refer to the next few pages for advice.

✓ All good? Then your item is a keeper!

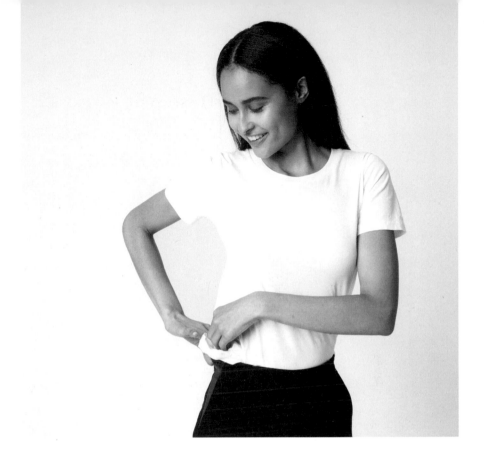

A word on alterations

For a small amount of money, a good tailor can improve the fit of many pieces with just a few tweaks and stitches.

One thing to note here is that some alterations are far trickier and therefore also more expensive than others. As a rule of thumb, taking something in is usually easier than letting it out. That's why the typical recommendation is that you buy the size that fits the larger part of your body well (your bust or hips for example), and get the rest taken in, either by having darts put in or the side seam adjusted. Also, shoulders and armholes are tricky in general, so it's best to go the extra mile and find pieces that fit you well in those areas and get the rest of the piece adjusted as necessary.

These are the top three easy alterations:

1. Shortening the hemlines of pants, skirt, dresses, tops, and sleeves
2. Adding darts to make a top, dress, or pair of pants slightly more fitted around the waist or bust
3. Taking in the side seams of skirts, dresses, tops, and sleeves (as long as you have enough room in the armhole)

Common fit problems and how to fix them

	PROBLEM	SOLUTION
PANTS		
Mirror check	The legs are too long.	Have a tailor hem the legs.
	The waistband feels uncomfortably tight and digs into your stomach.	Size up or find a pair with a higher rise.
	There's extra fabric that bunches up in the crotch area.	Try a pair of pants with a lower waistline.
	"Whiskers" in the crotch, groin area, or upper thighs.	Size up.
	Camel toe.	Try one size up. If that doesn't fix things, find a higher-waisted pair of pants.
	The pockets pop open.	Size up or get the pockets removed and sewn shut.
	The zipper gaps open at the top or slides down when you move.	Check if this happens with a bigger size too. If it does, it's a construction issue. Better skip this pair.
Movement check	The pants slip down as you walk (aka saggy-butt syndrome).	Find a pair with a higher rise that can hold onto your waist as an anchor. Or ask a tailor to add darts to the waistband.
	Your backside is on full display when you bend over or sit down.	Same as above: Choose a pair with a higher rise or get the waistband taken in.
	The pants feel super tight around the stomach or thighs when you sit down.	Size up. If your thighs feel fine and the only issue is a too-tight waistband, try a pair with a higher rise.
SKIRTS		
Mirror Check	The skirt is too long.	Get it hemmed.
	The fabric stretches and wrinkles across your thighs.	The skirt is too small for your hips. Pick one size up (get the waistband taken in if necessary).
	The waistband feels tight.	Size up or find a skirt with a higher waistline.
Movement Check	The skirt rides up as you walk.	The skirt is likely too small around the hips and thighs. Try a bigger size.
	The skirt shifts and rotates around your waist as you move.	Size down or have a tailor add darts to the waistband for a snugger fit.
	The skirt is so tight you can take only mini steps.	The skirt is either too small for you or poorly designed. Try a bigger size or just skip this model entirely.

	PROBLEM	SOLUTION

TOPS, SKIRTS, AND DRESSES

	PROBLEM	SOLUTION
Mirror Check	The piece feels tight around the bust but loose around the stomach (or the other way around).	Unless it's part of the design, tops should generally have a consistent fit throughout the torso. If your piece is too loose around the waist, you can have a tailor adjust the side seams or put in darts. If it's too loose around the chest, find a different style.
	Creases or pooled fabric next to the armpits, just above the bustline.	The piece may be poorly constructed or simply too small for you around the bustline. Try a bigger size to see if that improves things.
	For button-front blouses and shirts: the fabric pulls at the buttons or even gaps open in between.	This piece is too tight, so size up!
Movement Check	When you lift your arms, the torso of the piece moves up with them.	Try a bigger size. If that doesn't help, the armhole of this piece is set too low and might uncomfortably restrict your movements.
	The piece feels tight around your armpits, elbows, or wrists when you bend your arms and swirl them around.	Size up.
	The fabric around the shoulders bunches up when you cross your arms.	Size down.
	The piece feels tight around your shoulders when you cross your arms.	Size up.

JACKETS AND COATS

	PROBLEM	SOLUTION
Mirror Check	There is a dip in the fabric on the side of your arms just underneath the shoulder pads.	This is called a shoulder divot and happens when the shoulder pads extend past the shoulder of the wearer. It's a tell-tale sign that the piece is too big for you in the shoulders. Size down.
	The fabric is pulling and creasing around the shoulder seams.	Size up.
	The piece fits your shoulders well but is too loose around your waist.	Get it altered. A good tailor can take in the waistline of most jackets and coats by adding a few darts.
	The piece fits your shoulders well but sags around the chest area.	This piece is too big, but sizing up isn't an option because then it won't fit your shoulders anymore. Find a different piece altogether.
	The piece fits your shoulders well but won't button up.	Consider leaving the jacket or coat unbuttoned. If you want or need to be able to close it, buy the bigger size and have a tailor adjust the waist (and shoulders) as necessary.
Movement Check	When you lift your arms, the torso of the piece moves up with them.	Try a bigger size. If that doesn't help, the armhole of this piece is set too low and might uncomfortably restrict your movements.
	The upper back of this piece feels tight when you hug someone or bend over.	Size up.

21 / Maintaining and updating your wardrobe throughout the year: A timeline

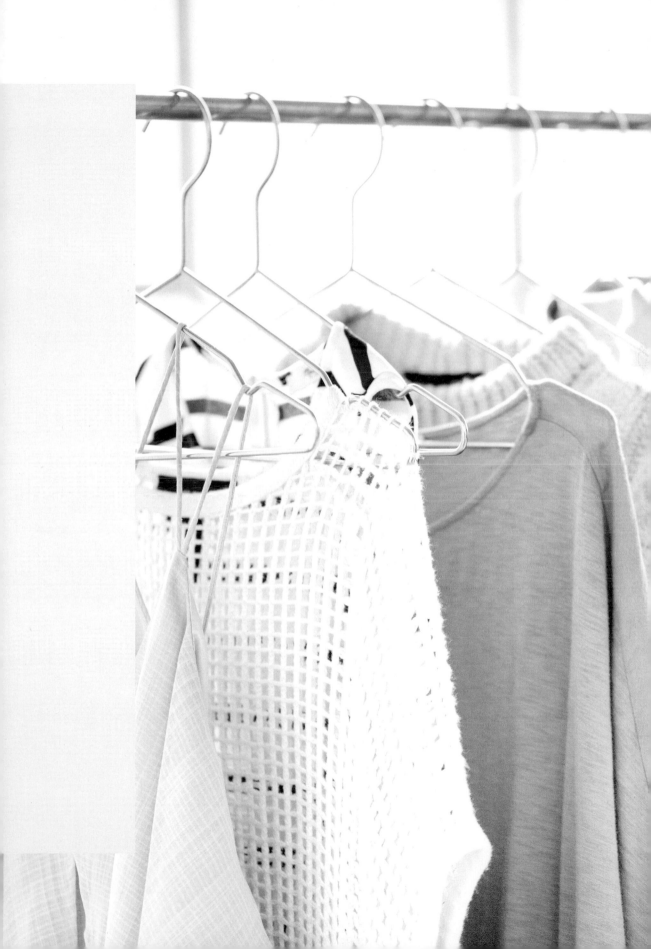

Here's a quick and easy guide to keeping your closet in great shape all year long and preparing your wardrobe for every new season through regular updates.

If you have worked through all the steps in this book until this point, you deserve a big pat on the back! You've discovered your personal style, you have built your dream wardrobe, and you have mastered the art of shopping (or at least you are well on your way!).

You've successfully completed closet bootcamp, so feel free to relish in that achievement and take your favorite new looks out to celebrate!

And when you come back, read through the next few pages to learn how to *maintain* your closet.

Because here's the thing: not even the most carefully curated wardrobe is ever 100 percent done. Your life isn't static, and neither is your personal style. Even if you love every single piece in your wardrobe right now, chances are that in a year or so you'll want to express a slightly different angle of your style, switch up one of your outfit formulas, or fall in love with new styles. Or perhaps you'll get a promotion, move to a new city, or take up rock climbing. A great closet is one that can grow and evolve alongside you, your style, and your life.

And that's why every wardrobe needs regular updates throughout the year, ideally at the beginning of every new season. Each update gives you the chance to take care of four basic maintenance tasks:

1. Preparing your wardrobe for the upcoming season
2. Redefining your personal style and incorporating a few new pieces, colors, or silhouettes into your look (optional)

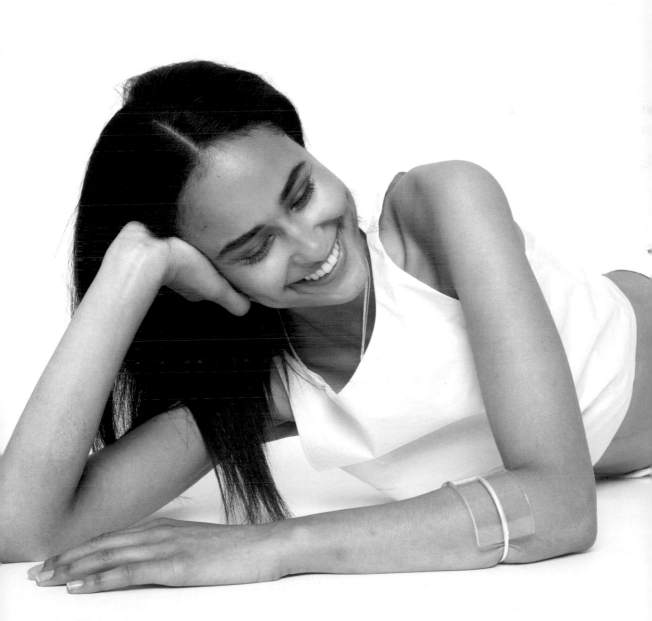

3. Making sure your wardrobe is well tailored to your lifestyle and your plans for the next few months
4. Dealing with repairs and replacing broken or worn-out wardrobe essentials

So what exactly does a wardrobe update look like and how often should you do one? Keep reading to find out!

When to update your wardrobe

My recommendation is that twice a year, just before fall and spring, you do a thorough seasonal overhaul. This is when you put off-season clothes into storage, review your personal style and lifestyle, map out your fall and spring wardrobe, and shop for a few new pieces if you like (skip to page 254 for a full list of steps). Seasonal overhauls are the meat and potatoes of your closet maintenance program.

In addition to seasonal overhauls, do a mini update twice a year to adjust your fall and spring wardrobe to the more extreme temperatures of the winter and summer seasons. That could mean checking your stock of scarves, gloves, winter coats, and thermal underwear if you live in a cold climate. Or it could mean buying another bikini and some sandals to prep for your summer holiday. Since you'll have done the bulk of wardrobe planning during your seasonal overhaul, mini updates should be quick and easy and take no more than a single shopping trip to complete.

The graphic on page 253 shows you a timeline for a yearly cycle of seasonal overhauls and mini updates. Keep in mind that this is just a sample; the ideal timing for each of your four wardrobe updates depends on the climate of where you live.

Here in Berlin, Germany, where I live, fall tends to start in October, winter in January, spring in April, and summer in July. I know how long it takes me to complete my seasonal overhauls (about two weeks) and mini updates (one afternoon), and from that I can deduce by what time of the year I should get started with each. The weather here also varies a lot between summer and winter, so for me, *cold-weather essentials* really does mean thermal underwear and chunky knit sweaters. But if you live in a milder climate, your idea of a winter wardrobe may simply mean switching to long sleeves and wearing tights with your skirts.

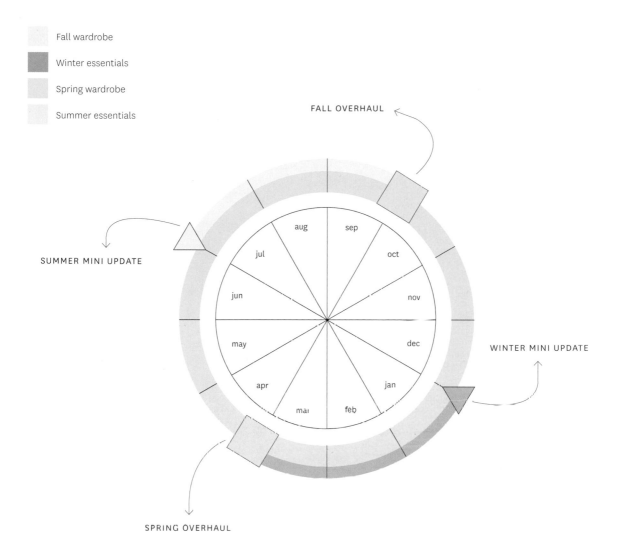

Fall wardrobe

Winter essentials

Spring wardrobe

Summer essentials

FALL OVERHAUL

SUMMER MINI UPDATE

WINTER MINI UPDATE

SPRING OVERHAUL

aug sep

jul oct

jun nov

may dec

apr jan

mar feb

If you live in a place where the weather stays relatively constant throughout the year, you may even be able to skip the mini updates entirely as well as the storage steps of the seasonal overhauls. But it's still a good idea to regularly revisit your wardrobe—at least every six months—to make sure it still fits your style and lifestyle and to deal with repairs.

And, of course, if you're located in the southern hemisphere, you'll be doing your fall overhaul in March or April and your spring overhaul in September or October.

Take a few minutes to sketch out your own cycle of seasonal overhauls and mini updates. When do your fall and spring wardrobes need to be ready, respectively? And when does winter and summer start where you live?

SEASONAL OVERHAULS

 Purpose: To prep your wardrobe for the upcoming season and keep it well-tailored to your style and lifestyle

When: Twice a year, once just before fall and once just before spring

Step 1: Move off season pieces into storage
Pack up everything that you won't be wearing during the next six months and put it into storage. Move seasonal pieces you had previously stored back into your closet.

Step 2: Create a seasonal style profile
Collect some fresh new inspiration and list any new colors, specific pieces, or styling tricks you want to try out this season. Then write a fall/winter version of your style profile. Optional: Put together a little mood board that matches your updated style profile.

Step 3: Detox your closet
Go through your closet and put anything that doesn't work with the style profile you just outlined into storage (or get rid of it entirely if you know you won't wear it again). Also deal with repairs and replacements.

Step 4: Review your lifestyle for the next season
Review your lifestyle for the next season. What activities will you need clothes for? Also note down any special occasions or trips. For fall, think family gatherings, holiday office parties, New Year's, and so on. For spring, think weddings, summer vacations, and so on.

Step 5: Give your wardrobe structure
Take a moment to figure out which color palette and outfit formulas you want to wear this season, as well as which types of key pieces, basics, and statement pieces would best reflect the overall look you are going for.

Step 6: Identify missing pieces

Based on the previous steps, write a detailed shopping list of every piece you still need to buy. Organize your list by priority.

Step 7: Shop as needed

Look for high-quality pieces that fit all your criteria and that you can see yourself wearing for seasons to come.

Step 8: Come up with some go-to looks

Experiment with your new seasonal wardrobe and put together a few new favorite outfits.

Step 9: Reorganize your closet

If necessary, rearrange your closet to reflect your new wardrobe structure.

MINI UPDATES

 Purpose: To adjust your fall and spring wardrobe for the more extreme temperatures of the winter and summer seasons

When: Twice a year, once just before winter and once just before summer

Step 1: Check your stock of cold- and warm-weather essentials

For winter: Do you have enough outerwear, gloves, hats, scarves, warm sweaters, winter boots, and other weather-appropriate pieces in storage or in your closet already?

For summer: Do you own enough bikinis, tops, shorts, summer dresses, sandals, and other summer essentials?

Step 2: Buy missing pieces

Write a shopping list beforehand.

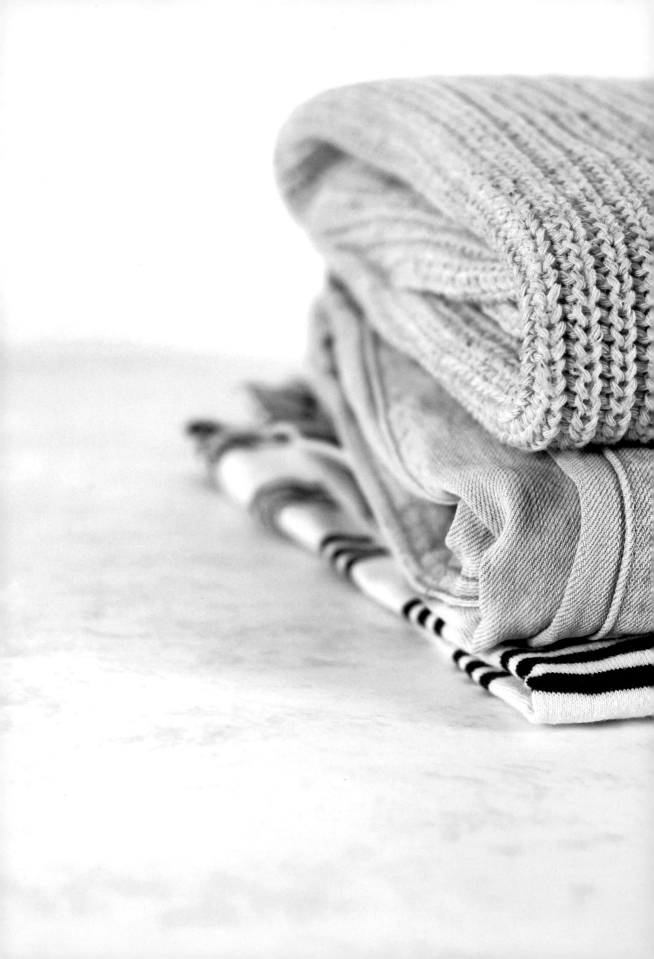

Conclusion

I hope this book has helped you explore your relationship to clothes, discover your unique likes and dislikes, and build a wardrobe that makes you feel confident and inspired everyday. And I hope you had a ton of fun along the way!

And remember: Even the most perfectly curated closet isn't meant to be static. Your style is ever evolving, just like you are.

So feel free to reread this book or repeat your favorite exercises whenever your wardrobe needs a little tweaking.

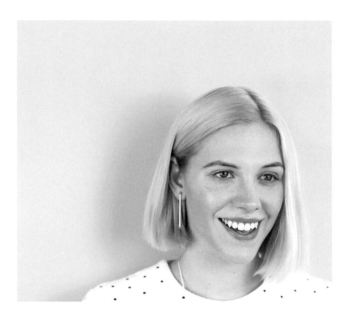

About the Author

Anuschka Rees is a writer and the founder of popular style blog INTO MIND. She lives in Berlin, Germany. *The Curated Closet* is her first book.

INTO-MIND.com
instagram.com/anuschkarees
facebook.com/intomind

Acknowledgments

Big thank yous go to Kaitlin Ketchum, Lindsay Edgecombe, Anna Rose Hankow, Margaux Keres, and Emma Campion for all their hard work and enthusiasm; to all the readers of INTO-MIND for their input and encouragement; and to Ben and my parents for their love and support.

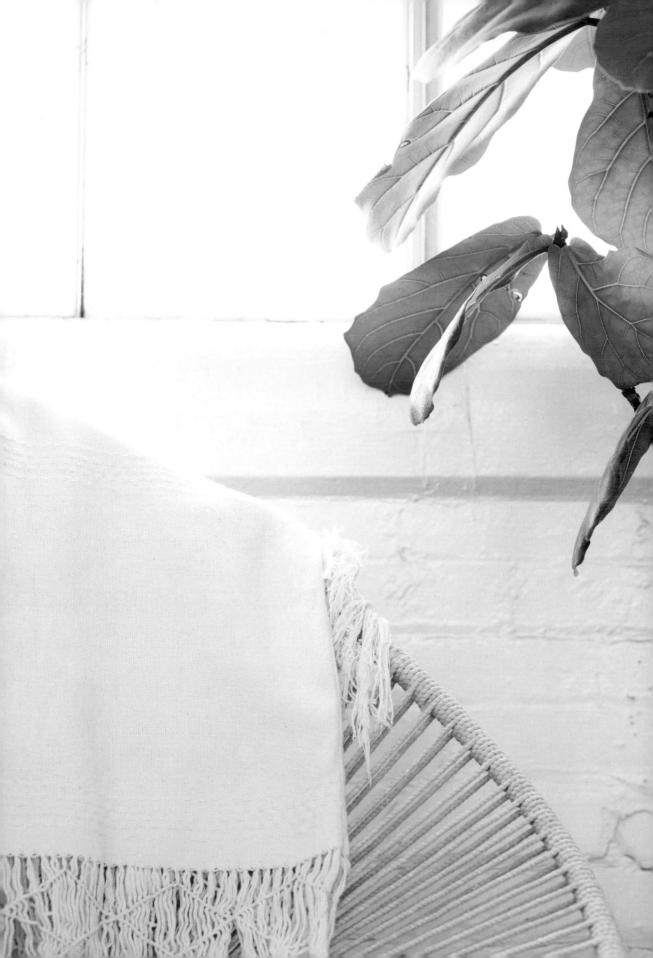

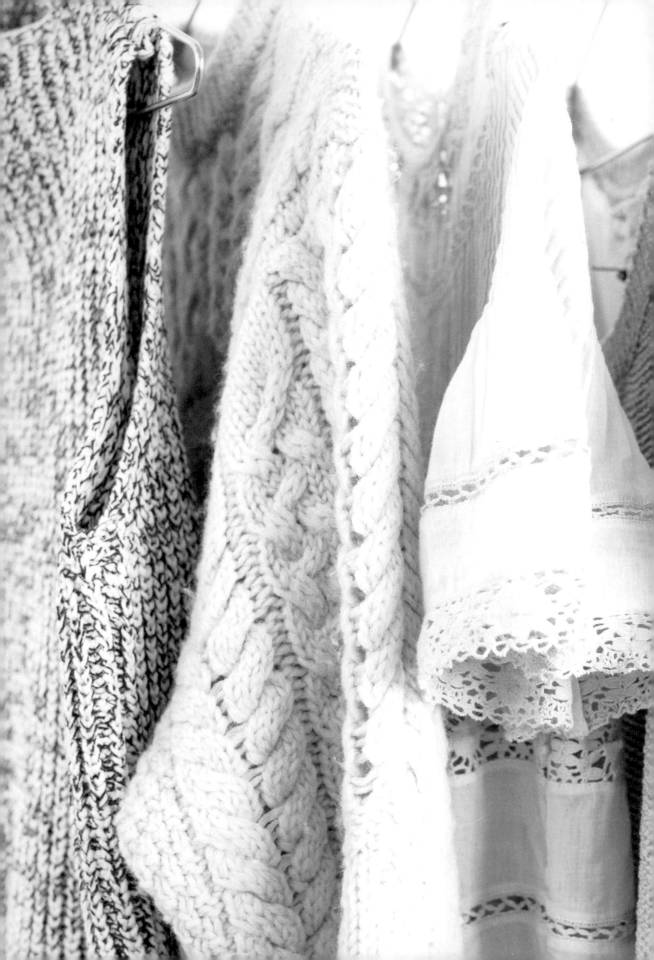

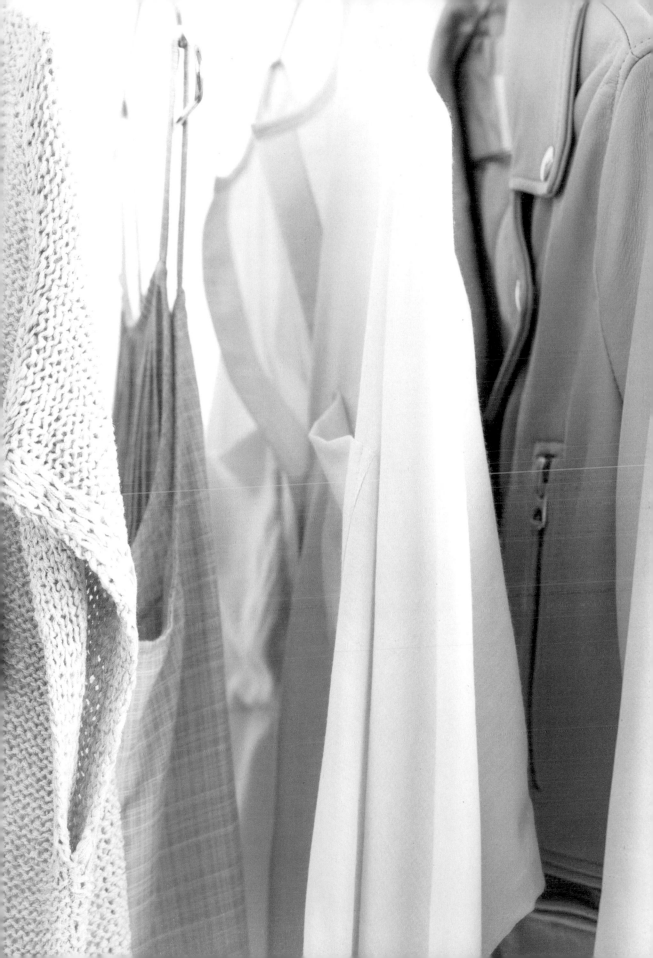

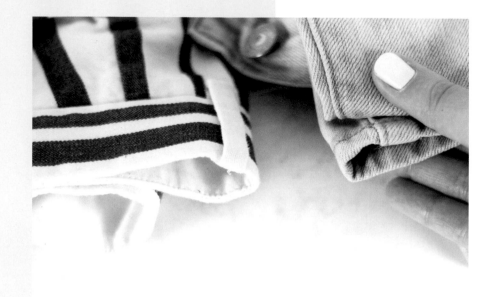

Index

Library of Congress Cataloging-in-Publication Data
Names: Rees, Anuschka, author.
Title: The curated closet : a simple system for discovering your personal
    style and building your dream wardrobe / by Anuschka Rees.
Description: First edition. | New York : Ten Speed Press, an imprint of the
    Crown Publishing Group, a division of Penguin Random House LLC, [2016] |
    Includes bibliographical references and index.
Identifiers: LCCN 2015046729 (print) | LCCN 2016000776 (ebook)
Subjects: LCSH: Fashion. | Clothing and dress. | Beauty, Personal.
Classification: LCC TX340 .R44 2016 (print) | LCC TX340 (ebook) | DDC
    646/.3—dc23
LC record available at http://lccn.loc.gov/2015046729

Trade Paperback ISBN: 978-1-60774-948-6
eBook ISBN: 978-1-60774-949-3

Printed in China

Design by Margaux Keres

Model photography styling by Alexandra Heckel
Clothing photography styling by Lisa Moir

10 9 8 7 6 5 4 3 2 1

First Edition